PROSTATE CANCER

A Patient's Guide to Treatment

Arthur Centeno, M.D. • Gary Onik, M.D.

Addicus Books
Omaha, Nebraska

An Addicus Nonfiction Book

ISBN# 1-886039-69-0
Cover design by George Foster
Illustrations by Jack Kusler

This book is not intended to serve as a substitute for a physician, nor is it the authors' intent to give medical advice contrary to that of an attending physician.

Library of Congress Cataloging-in-Publication Data

Centeno, Arthur, 1953-
 Prostate cancer : a patient's guide to treatment / Arthur Centeno, Gary Onik.
  p. cm.
Includes index.
ISBN 1-886039-69-0 (alk. paper)
1. Prostate—Cancer—Popular works. I. Onik, Gary, 1952- II. Title.

RC280.P7C46 2004
616.99'463—dc22   2004000036

Addicus Books, Inc.
P.O. Box 45327
Omaha, Nebraska 68145
www.AddicusBooks.com

Printed in the United States of America
10 9 8 7 6 5 4 3 2 1

To my late wife, Virginia, and to the memory of
my patients who have lost their battles with cancer.
They have taught me about the human spirit,
the will to live, and the dignity of fighting the good fight.
Arthur Centeno, M.D.

To the courageous patients who have advanced
our understanding and treatment of prostate cancer
by becoming part of our clinical trials over the past decade.
Gary Onik, M.D.

Contents

Acknowledgments

I would like to acknowledge Mary Campbell and Debbie Cooper, who have made this project fun, enjoyable, and most of all possible. I want to thank my partners, especially Johnny Reyna, M.D., Tom O'Neill, M.D., Ritchie Spence, M.D., and Andrew Tobon, M.D., who allow me to pursue an interest in prostate cancer. I want especially to thank the families of patients with prostate cancer for being there to help their husband, father, brother, or son through an emotionally tumultuous time. I want to thank my mom and dad for working so hard to help me become the person and physician that I am today. I want to thank Dawna Carr for always having a smile for me, in good times and bad.

Arthur Centeno, M.D.

I would like to acknowledge my wife, Janet, who has endured the ups and downs of a life tied to the performance of medical research; Dr. Allan Stam, who has been my friend and mentor throughout my medical career and who established for me the standards by which a medical career should be conducted; and the administration of Florida Hospital/Celebration Health who have supported so heartily our prostate cancer research program despite the financial burdens that it sometimes imposed.

Gary Onik, M.D.

Introduction

If you have been diagnosed with prostate cancer, you are not alone. Some 200,000 men are diagnosed with the disease annually in the United States. As you may already know, a diagnosis of cancer is the beginning of a journey that none of us would choose to take. It is a journey that most of us begin with fear and trepidation. But thanks to modern medicine, many of our fears can be put to rest. Much can be done to fight prostate cancer. And that fight is often won, especially when the cancer is diagnosed early.

Having treated thousands of patients, we have learned that one of the ways a patient can combat fear and anxiety is to become an active participant in his treatment. This means learning about the disease and the treatment options. The more you know, the less you face the unknown. Knowledge helps take away some of the fear.

It is our hope that this book will help you make smart decisions and take responsibility for managing prostate cancer and its treatment. No book, however complete, can substitute for your doctor's expertise and advice. But with the information on these pages and in the scores of other excellent resources for prostate cancer patients and their loved ones, you can be an active partner in the disease's management and possibly in its cure.

In today's health care environment, it's more important than ever for patients to be well informed. For one thing, the pace of research has accelerated and new discoveries are almost as accessible to the health care consumer as to the medical profession. Highly motivated patients can access the Internet and, with just a little detective work, can find a world of information and support.

On the other hand, managed care has changed the health care landscape. Some doctors feel pressured to see more patients and spend less time with each one. That places more responsibility on you to learn as much as you can about your condition and whatever solutions are available.

Even though a cancer diagnosis is alarming, there's a certain amount of power that comes with it—call it the "prostate cancer patient's bill of rights."

- You do *not* have the right to remain silent. Make all the noise you can if it helps you get the information and care you need.
- You have the right to feel bewildered, alone, afraid, depressed, and angry.
- You have the right to get professional help if negative emotions overwhelm you and keep you from acting in your own best interest.
- You have the right to get a second opinion ... or a third ... or more, if necessary.
- Your have the right to seek support from family, friends, medical professionals, prostate cancer patients, spiritual advisers, and others who can help.
- You have the right to make your own decisions about treatment.
- You have the right to trust your instincts as well as your knowledge.
- You have the right *and* the ability to understand your disease and take as much time as you need to gather information and support.

- Perhaps best of all, you have the right to become a mentor to others who are reeling from the news that they, too, have prostate cancer.

Keep these rights in mind as you begin your journey. You will find empowerment.

*In the depths of winter I finally learned
that there was in me an invincible summer.*
—Albert Camus
1913–1960

The Prostate and Prostate Cancer

"**Y**es, you have prostate cancer."

If you, or someone you love, have heard these words spoken, your first reaction might well have been panic, numbness, despair, or a combination of these feelings. Many people experience a dizzying whirl of emotions after receiving a cancer diagnosis—anger, depression, concern for family and loved ones, fear of the unknown, and sometimes a nameless dread that comes and goes in those first days and weeks.

All this is natural and normal. In some ways your life will never be the same. You'd be less than human if you didn't grieve, at least briefly, for the loss of your "old" life.

Even so—though you might find this hard to believe right now—there are thousands and thousands of prostate cancer survivors who will tell you the diagnosis was one of the best things that ever happened to them. Once they got over the initial shock and started looking for answers and finding support, they saw life as the wonderful gift it truly is. They educated themselves about the disease and the many ways of dealing with it. They discovered that knowledge is power and learned to use that power for their own health and well-being. They forged new relationships, strengthened existing ones, and shared— perhaps for the first time—their deepest feelings and greatest fears.

Through this process, these survivors learned that prostate cancer is curable—yes, *curable*—when found in the early stages. And they saw how their own decisions and actions could help them stay healthy for many years to come.

The Prostate Gland

To better understand prostate cancer, let's first examine the role of the prostate gland itself. The *prostate* is a muscular gland about the size and shape of a walnut. Part of the urinary and reproductive systems, it is located in the pelvis below the urinary bladder and sits just in front of the rectum. The *urethra*, which carries urine and semen out of the body through the penis, runs through the prostate like a straw through a doughnut hole.

Because it is actually several small glands encased in the *prostate capsule,* the prostate is sometimes described as having two lobes, three lobes, or several zones. Of these, the *peripheral zone*, or outer zone, where most prostate cancer begins, is the largest; the muscular *central zone* prevents semen from backing up into the bladder during ejaculation; and the *transition zone*, which surrounds the urethra, is the only site for a common noncancerous disorder called *benign prostatic hyperplasia (BPH)*.

Prostate Gland

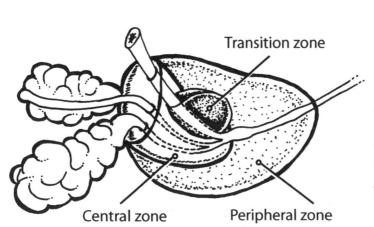

Transition zone

Central zone

Peripheral zone

Prostate Gland Side View

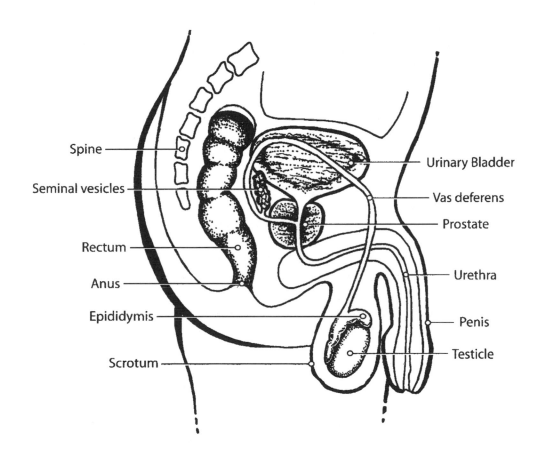

Prostate Gland Frontal View

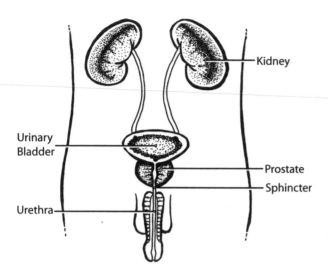

Kidney

Urinary Bladder

Prostate

Sphincter

Urethra

The Prostate and Reproduction

Your prostate gland is small but mighty. It weighs between 20 and 40 grams. By comparison, a first class letter weighs 30 grams. Small as it is, the prostate is essential for normal human reproduction. It adds important fluid and nutrients to sperm during ejaculation. Among these nutrients are citric acid, potassium, calcium, and zinc.

To function properly, the prostate depends on male hormones *(androgens)*, chiefly *testosterone.* Testosterone is responsible for the traits usually associated with men—body hair, deep voice, musculature, and so on. The prostate converts testosterone to another, more potent male hormone, *dihydrotestosterone* or *DHT.*

Of course, the prostate alone does not fuel the reproductive process. The *testicles* or *testes* manufacture sperm and most of the testosterone upon which the prostate depends. The *adrenal glands* also produce small amounts of androgens. A small gland, the *epididymis*, sits next to the testes, and stores sperm until they mature.

Just before the male orgasm, numerous muscles work together to produce semen and pump it out of the body. These muscles squeeze *seminal fluid* from the prostate and from the adjacent *seminal vesicles* through small pores into the urethra, where two 18-inch tubes called *vasa deferentia* deposit sperm. The vasa deferentia and the ducts of the seminal vesicles join in the prostate to form the *ejaculatory duct.* During ejaculation, sperm and seminal fluid—the components of semen—travel through the urethra and exit the penis.

The Prostate and Urination

Prostate illness can interfere with your ability to urinate and in some cases can damage your kidneys and other urinary tract structures. Because the prostate surrounds the urethra, prostate enlargement can squeeze and eventually choke the urethra and make simple urination an agonizing chore.

The urinary tract begins at the *kidneys*, located at the base of the ribs on either side of the spine. These amazing organs are the body's main filters, cleansing impurities from about 45 gallons of water every day. Most of this water is recirculated through the body, producing only two quarts of waste, in the form of urine, in most men.

Do as much research as you can. Proceed deliberately but without rushing. Choose the best doctor you can find. Go with your best gut instinct and then never look back.
—John, 61

Urine travels to the *urinary bladder* through tubes called *ureters*. The bladder, located above the prostate, holds about a pint of urine. It empties into the urethra, which carries it through a muscle called the *urinary sphincter* and out through the penis. The urinary sphincter is responsible for continence, your ability to contain the flow of urine.

For this marvelous internal cleansing system to help you stay healthy, every mechanism must be in working order. Prostate disorders can harm this delicate balance and keep the structures of the urinary tract from doing their jobs.

Noncancerous Prostate Disorders

While we're discussing the urination process, let's examine two common noncancerous prostate conditions that can interfere with urination. These conditions are benign prostatic hyperplasia and prostatitis. These conditions usually do not affect younger men, but often develop after a man has reached his 40s. It is important to note that these two conditions do not cause prostate cancer, nor do they place you at greater risk for it.

Benign Prostatic Hyperplasia

Benign prostatic hyperplasia (BPH) is an enlarged prostate. The enlargement comes from small noncancerous (benign) growths (hyperplasia) inside the prostate. In a man with BPH, the prostate might grow from the normal walnut size to apricot size after age 40 and lemon size by age 60.

As the prostate grows, it squeezes the urethra and makes it difficult to pass urine. BPH symptoms include urinary irregularities—frequent or urgent urination, a weak urinary stream, or difficulty urinating, for example. Even so, only about half of men with BPH require treatment.

Sometimes, however, symptoms become more than a nuisance. If the bladder is unable to empty properly, urine can back up into the kidneys and impair their essential function, straining impurities from body fluids.

There are drugs on the market for treatment of BPH, but many doctors believe that medication is just a stopgap measure that postpones the inevitable. When BPH is severe, surgery may be needed, usually *transurethral resection of the prostate (TURP),* which requires no skin incision. Surgeons remove the overgrown prostate tissue with an instrument attached to a slender tube that is inserted through the urethra.

Prostatitis

Prostatitis is inflammation of the prostate. Its symptoms include frequent, difficult, or painful urination. Other symptoms include pain in joints, muscles, the lower back, and the pelvis; pain during ejaculation; aches, fever, chills, and blood in the urine.

Acute bacterial prostatitis, caused by bacteria, afflicts many men between 40 and 60 years of age. *Chronic bacterial prostatitis,* different from the acute form by being recurrent and longer lasting, is more often found in men between 50 and 80. Bacterial forms of prostatitis are sometimes referred to as prostate infections.

Nonbacterial prostatitis, which is of unknown cause, occurs most often in men from 30 to 50. Though antibiotics are usually effective against bacterial prostatitis, the nonbacterial form has no known cure. Like arthritis and other chronic ailments, however, nonbacterial prostatitis is treatable with anti-inflammatory drugs.

Prostate Cancer

Cancer is a collection of cells that are growing out of control. How does this happen? Healthy cells have predictable growth limits and life spans. Not only do cancer cells grow past normal limits, they don't die when they're supposed to. Instead, they divide and spread, sometimes uncontrollably.

For me, one of the joys of having been through this cancer journey has been reaching out to other guys and their mates and sharing my experiences, offering them hope for a successful recovery such as I have had.
— Fletch, 49

A mass of cancer cells is called a *tumor,* but not all tumors are cancerous. A *benign* tumor might grow and squeeze nearby organs, but it does not spread in an aggressive or life-threatening way. Cancer cells, however, can break away from a primary *malignant* tumor site and spread, or *metastasize,* to nearby organs or to distant sites through blood or lymph vessels. Cancer destroys normal tissue and creates new tumors as it spreads.

How does cancer spread through the lymph system? *Lymph* is a fluid that bathes every living cell in the body. You sometimes see this clear fluid escaping when you skin your knee, for example. Lymph fights cancer by draining waste from cells, carrying it through vessels and into lymph nodes, which filter the fluid and remove harmful substances. Sometimes, however, there are more cancer cells than the lymph nodes can handle, and the lymph vessels themselves become vehicles for spreading cancer.

Prostate cancer has recently overtaken skin cancer as the most common cancer among men in the United States. More than 200,000 men, or one out of six, are diagnosed with prostate cancer in the United States every year. As many as five million Americans are living with prostate cancer right now. It kills more men than any cancer except lung cancer.

However, not all cancers offer the potential for cure that prostate cancer does. And of more than 100 types of cancer that occur in the United States, prostate cancer is comparatively slow growing. Many men with *microscopic prostate cancer* never know they have it and eventually die from unrelated causes. In fact, most men with prostate cancer do not die from prostate cancer.

Some men with elevated PSAs think they don't have prostate cancer because they "feel fine." I tell every man who will listen, including my sons, that by the time they no longer feel fine it may be too late for a cure.
— Newt, 67

This doesn't mean you should ignore symptoms or delay seeking treatment, however. Untreated, prostate cancer can spread within the prostate capsule and outward to seminal vesicles, lymph nodes, bones, lungs, liver, and elsewhere in the body.

Typically, prostate cancer starts in the peripheral zone of the gland. Male hormones, especially testosterone, stimulate growth of both normal and cancerous cells in the prostate. Accordingly, testosterone fuels prostate cancer growth.

Symptoms of Prostate Cancer

Early prostate cancer has no symptoms. You could be feeling hale and hearty when you are diagnosed. For many men, the diagnosis comes as a complete surprise. Malignant tumors in the prostate generally start out very small. It usually takes years for prostate cancers to grow large enough to obstruct the flow of urine. Fortunately, modern diagnostic methods can detect prostate cancer long before symptoms have a chance to develop.

If prostate cancer grows enough to exhibit symptoms, they are much like those of noncancerous prostate disorders. One or more of the following symptoms can indicate prostate cancer:

- Getting up at night to urinate
- Frequent urination during the day
- Weak or interrupted urinary flow
- Difficulty starting the urine stream
- Dribbling
- Urgency
- Leakage
- Pain or burning during urination
- Needing to strain to urinate
- Less rigid erections than normal
- Pain during ejaculation
- Less ejaculate (semen) than normal
- Impotence

Though such symptoms may not indicate prostate cancer, they should never be ignored. Almost any disease, no matter how minor it is in the beginning, can be dangerous if left untreated.

Prostate cancer that has spread beyond the gland itself can cause a range of symptoms, depending on where the cancer is located. Such symptoms include pain, sometimes intermittent, in the back, ribs, hip, or shoulder; fatigue; weakness; and generalized aches and pains.

Even though these symptoms are vague and could easily be harmless, don't ignore them. Too many men regard their symptoms, whether difficulty urinating or intermittent aches and pains, as "normal signs of aging." It bears repeating: See your doctor right away if you're experiencing symptoms you can't easily explain.

Risk Factors for Prostate Cancer

All men are at risk for prostate cancer. The incidence of the disease is strongly related to age. Because men typically live longer than their fathers and grandfathers did, prostate cancer diagnoses are on the rise. Other risk factors include the following:

- **Family history**. New research indicates that a family history of prostate cancer or breast cancer, especially before the age of 50, greatly increases the risk of early prostate cancer in men and early breast cancer in women. Doctors recommend earlier annual screenings starting at age 40 rather than 50 for those at risk for prostate cancer.

- **Race and ethnicity**. African American men are at higher risk for prostate cancer than any other group worldwide. No one is sure why this is the case, though some researchers think that since dark skin absorbs less sunlight, the body produces less vitamin D, which protects against prostate cancer. Other scientists speculate that differences in diet may play a role. Hispanic men are also at higher risk than Caucasians in the United States. Like men with a family history of prostate or breast cancer, African American and Hispanic men should have annual prostate screenings starting at age 40.

- **Location and environment**. Worldwide, prostate cancer is more deadly in areas of lowest ultraviolet radiation. Prostate cancer death rates are highest in Sweden and Canada. Interestingly, Japanese men are at lowest risk. After these men move to the United States, however, their risk rises quickly, which indicates that diet and environment may be powerful risk factors.

    In the United States, men at highest risk are those who

live in the northwest, the Rocky Mountain states, New England, the north-central states, and the south Atlantic states. Again, no one is sure why this is the case, but explanations proposed include environmental pollution and traditional diet.

- **Occupation**. Though the evidence is inconclusive, it appears that farmers, mechanics, and welders are at higher risk than the general population. In the case of farmers, exposure to pesticides and other chemicals may subject them to enough "insults" at the cellular level to cause cells to mutate and become cancerous. Mechanics and welders may be vulnerable because of exposure to the element cadmium, which interferes with zinc absorption. Men with prostate cancer tend to have lower levels of zinc in their bodies.

- **Other possible risk factors**. There is weak evidence that smoking may raise the level of hormones that fuel prostate cancer growth. Men who have had vasectomies are probably not at higher risk, though some researchers have suggested such a link.

Most researchers now believe that a combination of heredity and environment is responsible for most prostate cancers.

Preventing Prostate Cancer

For more than a decade, scientists have known that a high-fat, low-fiber diet greatly increases the likelihood of prostate cancer. Over and over, research has shown that a more healthful diet not only decreases the likelihood of prostate cancer, it may slow the cancer's growth. A southern Mediterranean diet emphasizing olive oil and cooked vegetables or a rural Japanese diet—high in rice, fish, soy, vegetables, and green tea—may actually prevent prostate cancer and help prevent recurrences.

Why is this the case? High dietary fat levels, especially from red meat and dairy products, may stimulate cancer cell growth or block mechanisms that protect cells from cancer. Another theory is that excess fat stimulates male hormone production.

Many doctors recommend that, whether or not you have prostate cancer, your diet include no more than 20 percent of its calories from fat. Most people—apart from those with allergies, food sensitivities, or other health problems with their own sets of dietary rules—will benefit from a variety of wholesome foods, including:

- **Soy products**, such as tofu and soy milk, which may block *angiogenesis*, the process by which cancer cells create blood vessels on which to travel through the body.

- **Green tea**, which contains *antioxidants* that neutralize cancer-causing *oxidants*, or *free radicals,* in the body.

- **Red grapes, grape juice, and red wine**, which also contain antioxidants, though of a different type than those in green tea.

- **Fresh fruits and vegetables**, which may contain *beta-carotene* (which protects against rapid cell growth), *lycopene* (an anticancer pigment present in red-colored foods), and antioxidants. In general, the darker the color, the greater the benefit. That gives you a lot of delicious, nourishing foods to choose from, including dark green leafy vegetables (spinach, romaine lettuce, and other salad greens), cruciferous vegetables (broccoli and cauliflower), beets, carrots, yams, strawberries, raspberries, blueberries, peas, watermelon, and citrus fruits.

- **Fresh herbs**, including oregano, peppermint, rosemary, and thyme, which contain antioxidants.

In most cases, you should try to get your nutrition from fresh foods, except meat, eggs, and seafood, which should be thoroughly cooked. Here are a few other exceptions:

- **Cooked tomatoes**, in the form of tomato paste, sauce, or juice, contain more lycopene than fresh tomatoes.

- **Vitamin E and selenium supplements** provide essential nutrients lacking in most diets. Both boost the immune system and fight free radicals. Don't take vitamin E supplements if you have a bleeding problem or you're taking blood thinners, and stop taking it several weeks before surgery or a biopsy. A safe selenium dose is about 200 micrograms per day.

If you take a multivitamin, check for levels of these nutrients; you might already be getting the recommended amounts. Recent studies have promoted calcium supplements for men as well as women, but excess calcium may block the body's production of vitamin D. Consult your doctor before taking these and any other supplements, and ask for recommended dosages in light of prescription and nonprescription drugs you are taking.

If you exercise regularly, keep it up; if you don't, ask your doctor to recommend an exercise plan. Besides its many other benefits,

---

Prostate Cancer Statistics

- 89% of men diagnosed with prostate cancer survive at least 5 years.

- 63% survive at least 10 years.

- 60% of diagnosed prostate cancers are still confined to the prostate.

- The 5-year relative survival rate for men with localized prostate cancer is 100%.

- 31% of prostate cancers are diagnosed after they have spread to tissues near the prostate. The 5-year survival rate for these men is 94%.

- Among the 11% of men whose prostate cancer has spread to distant parts of the body at the time of diagnosis, about 31% are expected to survive at least 5 years.

exercise is known to boost the immune system and improve mood and mental balance.

Men who exercise sensibly, don't smoke or drink excessive amounts of alcohol, and eat healthfully, might be less vulnerable to prostate cancer than less active men who smoke, drink heavily, and eat a lot of animal fat. The National Cancer Institute is sponsoring numerous prostate cancer prevention trials, which promise to reveal much more about the role of diet and lifestyle in prostate cancer.

2

Getting a Diagnosis

I f you've been putting off your annual physical or postponing that free prostate screening, don't delay any longer. If found early, prostate cancer is curable, but tends to become more aggressive as it grows.

A variety of diagnostic tests can help your doctor determine whether you have prostate cancer. Before prostate cancer screening and early detection were available, up to a third of first-time diagnoses found advanced prostate cancer. Today, advanced disease is involved in only about 5 percent of initial diagnoses. Simply put, screening and early detection are lifesavers.

Diagnostic Tests

To screen for prostate cancer, doctors first rely on a digital rectal examination (DRE) and a blood test that measures prostate-specific antigen (PSA). The American Cancer Society recommends annual DRE and PSA blood tests for men 50 and older. Some prostate cancer advocacy groups recommend annual exams beginning at age 45. African-American men and any man with a family history of prostate or breast cancer should have annual DRE and PSA blood tests starting at age 40.

Digital Rectal Exam

Though the *digital rectal exam (DRE)* is only a starting place, it often finds growths and other irregularities that might indicate cancer many years before you would notice any other symptoms. The exam may be slightly uncomfortable, but is very brief and seldom painful.

To perform a DRE, your doctor will insert a gloved, lubricated finger into the rectum. He or she will feel through the back rectal wall for lumps, enlargement, or hard, coarse, jagged, or uneven areas of the prostate that might indicate cancer or another prostatic disease. The healthy prostate is soft, smooth, and symmetrical, and there is a groove down the middle. If the doctor cannot feel the prostate's groove, the gland is probably enlarged. This and other abnormalities could be caused by previous prostate surgery or biopsy, past or present infections, or even stones in the prostate, as well as BPH, benign prostatic hyperplasia, a noncancerous enlargement. Or it could be prostate cancer.

Digital Rectal Exam

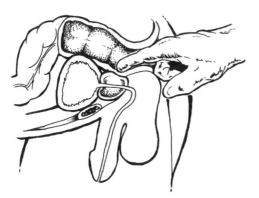

A normal prostate gland is soft and smooth. Most prostate cancers start in the outer "zone" of the prostate gland, and doctors are often able to feel lumps or other changes in the gland when performing a digital rectal exam (DRE).

The location of abnormalities is important. Growths due to BPH tend to be in the central gland, but almost three-fourths of prostate cancers start in the peripheral or outer zone, the area closest to the rectum. At least a fourth of prostate cancers, however, begin where the doctor can't reach. That's why the PSA blood test is so important; it often reveals prostate cancer that's not apparent in the DRE.

Some experts suggest that you go to the same doctor each year for your DRE, since, in theory at least, that doctor will be more likely to notice palpable changes in your prostate from year to year. If your primary care doctor isn't extremely well informed about prostate cancer or doesn't do rectal examinations, you might prefer to see a *urologist,* a doctor who has special knowledge of the male and female urinary tract and the male reproductive organs.

Prostate-Specific Antigen

Perhaps the screening test you've heard about most often is one which measures prostate-specific antigen, PSA; these antigens are *biomarkers,* also called *tumor markers,* and are normal substances in blood, other fluids, or tissues whose fluctuations sometimes indicate cancer. Think of a biomarker as similar to the measurement marks on your car's dipstick. There's a normal level of oil in your car's engine, just as there are normal levels of the various biomarkers in your body. If you check your car's oil level regularly, you know that a small decrease is probably normal, but a big drop means trouble, like a major leak. Checking the oil helps you find problems before there are symptoms, such as alarming knocks or pings from the engine or a blown gasket.

Likewise, checking patients' biomarkers helps doctors spot trouble before symptoms appear. Prostate cancer has several biomarkers. The most important is the protein called *PSA, prostate-specific antigen.* If there is a lot of PSA in your bloodstream, it usually means there's some type of prostate disorder. If the PSA level rises quickly over two or three tests, it can indicate a large or fast-growing tumor.

All prostate cells, both normal and cancerous, produce PSA. Small amounts of PSA normally enter the bloodstream. Cancerous cells, however, multiply more quickly than normal cells, and therefore, more PSA is produced. So an elevated PSA is a warning that something may be wrong and that more studies are needed. That "something" could be BPH, an inflammation or infection; a recent biopsy, catheterization, bladder surgery, or another procedure; or recent activity that "massages" the prostate, such as riding a bicycle or motorcycle. Sexual intercourse can elevate your PSA by as much as 10 percent. So that a temporary rise in your PSA doesn't throw off the test results, ask your doctor well in advance what you should do, and not do, to prepare.

If your DRE is normal but your PSA is mildly elevated, your doctor will ask for a urine sample to see if you have a prostate infection. If you do, the doctor will probably prescribe an antibiotic and do another PSA blood test several weeks after you've finished taking the medicine.

If prostatitis is not causing the elevated PSA, your doctor will want to recheck your PSA level two to six weeks later. If it is still elevated, further tests are called for, usually ultrasound and a prostate biopsy.

What Is a Normal PSA Level?

PSA is measured in *nanograms* per liter of blood. A nanogram is so small, one-billionth of a gram, that a very sensitive test is needed to detect it.

A normal PSA level is not the same for everyone. It varies, depending on age and ethnicity.

Age	Normal PSA	African American Normal PSA
40-50	2.5 or lower	2.0 or lower
50-60	3.5 or lower	3.0 or lower
60-70	4.5 or lower	4.0 or lower
70 and up	6.5 or lower	6.0 or lower

Not all the experts agree on these guidelines. Some say anything above 4.0 is suspicious regardless of the patient's age. Others advise men to have more studies if the first-time PSA is 2.0 or above.

Conditions other than prostate cancer can cause PSA levels to rise. Scientists have found several ways to interpret PSA test results to form a better idea of whether cancer is causing the PSA increase. One of these is called *PSA velocity (PSAV),* which compares PSA levels over time to see how quickly they are rising. Your doctor may suspect prostate cancer if your PSA rises by more than three-fourths of a nanogram per year.

Your doctor may also refer to *free PSA*, when interpreting your PSA scores. PSA is found in two forms in the blood: either it is attached to a protein or it is not attached, called "free." Patients who have more free PSA in their blood are less likely to have prostate cancer.

Transrectal Ultrasound

If the DRE or PSA indicates you might have prostate cancer, you'll probably have at least two additional diagnostic procedures, a *transrectal ultrasound (TRUS)* and a needle biopsy. Don't worry if these tests are scheduled several weeks after your checkup. Prostate cancer usually progresses slowly, allowing time to run the tests and do the studies that give very important information about the cancer. The more specific that information, the better you and your doctor can choose precisely the right treatment if cancer is found.

Men with prostate cancer should get a second and even a third opinion. I consulted another urologist and a radiation oncologist. All supported the radical prostatectomy route based on my age and my cancer's high Gleason score (8).

— Bill, 47

For the TRUS procedure, the doctor will insert a lubricated ultrasound probe into the rectum just behind the prostate. Because ultrasound waves bounce off normal tissue differently than off malignant tissue, the TRUS probe creates a picture of the prostate and abnormalities it might contain. The doctor views the picture on a TV screen.

TRUS shows the size of the prostate, an important baseline measurement, but it can't see all types of tumors. Some prostate tumors are distinct lumps, which often show up on TRUS, but other prostate tumors are spread out, and TRUS seldom shows these. As a result, a normal ultrasound could merely mean that you, like most men with prostate cancer, have lesions that are flat or small and scattered (*diffuse*). Like the DRE, transrectal ultrasound can be uncomfortable, though sedation is rarely needed.

Needle Biopsy

In a *needle biopsy*, a sample of body tissue is removed with a needle. This procedure can find cancer that a TRUS might miss. Many doctors do TRUS and a biopsy at the same time. They use the TRUS images on the TV screen to show them where to direct the biopsy needle. This makes the procedure more accurate than was possible when doctors had no guidance other than what they could feel with their fingers.

My family doctor didn't want to do the PSA and DRE when I was 45, so I asked for a referral to a urologist. My PSA was 5+ and there was cancer in the needle biopsy. I had surgery two years ago and my PSA is now undetectable. My twin brother is having prostate cancer surgery next month. Insist on the testing.
— *Jim, 48*

With the ultrasound probe in place, the doctor can direct the biopsy needle to suspicious areas. Using a high-speed biopsy "gun"—a long, thin, hollow, spring-loaded needle inserted through the ultrasound probe—the doctor removes several, usually 8 to 12, small cores of suspicious tissue. A *pathologist*, a physician who specializes in diagnosing diseases, examines these tissues under a microscope. The pathologist calculates the presence and amount of cancer, its *grade* (how much it deviates from normal tissue), and how advanced it appears to be.

Sometimes after these procedures, doctors are still unsure whether cancer is present and you'll need to repeat the TRUS and biopsy. If the pathologist is uncertain about the biopsy samples, ask your doctor about sending them to a pathologist who specializes in prostate biopsies.

Saturation Biopsies or 3D Global Mapping Biopsies

If a needle biopsy does not result in the discovery of cancer, but your physician still strongly suspects it, he or she may recommend a newer type of biopsy called a *saturation biopsy* or *3D global mapping biopsy.* This biopsy method is more extensive and systematic than the transrectal biopsy in which the needle is inserted through the rectum. For a saturation biopsy, the needle is guided by ultrasound technology and is inserted through the *perineum*, the area between the scrotum and the rectum. Watching on a television monitor, the physician can view the needle's path as it enters the prostate gland. Then, each tissue sample is labeled, according to which part of the gland it was taken from. This makes it possible to construct an exact "map" of the cancer's location.

Research shows that prostate cancer is found in 40 percent of men who have saturation biopsies after having at least three previously negative biopsies.

Preparing for a Biopsy

Your doctor will likely give you instructions prior to your biopsy. For at least a week before your biopsy, avoid alcohol and don't take any medicines or food supplements that can thin your blood and interfere with its ability to clot. These substances can include aspirin, ibuprofen (Motrin or Advil), and other nonsteroid anti-inflammatory drugs (except Tylenol), food supplements containing vitamin E, fish oil, ginkgo biloba, garlic, and the blood thinner Coumadin. At the time the biopsy is arranged, be sure to tell your doctor what prescription and over-the-counter medications and food supplements you're taking.

Most patients tolerate biopsy procedures well, but if you know you have a low pain threshold, talk with your doctor about ways to relieve any pain or discomfort during the biopsy. Don't feel timid about requesting one of the topical or local pain relievers available for this purpose. If you wish to be given intravenous sedation to make you sleep during the procedure, you will likely need to have the procedure performed in an outpatient surgery center.

After the Biopsy

TRUS and prostate biopsies are generally outpatient procedures. After having them, you'll probably be sore, so it's a good idea to arrange for someone to drive you home. The next day you can do just about anything you feel up to. You'll continue to take antibiotics, so don't drink alcohol during that time. The biopsy results should be available within two or three days.

If these tests show you have prostate cancer, you'll understandably be eager to start treatment. Many patients see their cancer as an enemy to be wiped out at the earliest possible moment. Taking a bit more time to study your cancer, however, is to your benefit. The more you and your doctor know, the better you can decide on the most effective treatment.

At this point, your doctor will investigate your cancer's *stage*, how far it has spread, and the *grade*, how aggressive the cancer is.

Biopsy Risks

Serious side effects from biopsies are rare. Some patients worry that a biopsy could cause the cancer to spread. This possibility is so remote that it should not prevent your having a biopsy.

Severe bleeding or infection occurs less than 1 percent of the time. It's normal to find blood in your urine, semen, or stool for a few weeks after a prostate biopsy.

Very rarely, infection after a prostate biopsy becomes serious, moving into the bloodstream and causing a high fever, shaking, and chills. This reaction, called *sepsis,* is a medical emergency. To reduce the risk of infection, your doctor will prescribe antibiotics, and you'll have a cleansing enema before the procedure.

Another rare but serious biopsy complication is a urinary blockage, indicated by pain and the inability to pass urine. Seek medical help immediately if you experience symptoms of infection or urinary blockage.

Staging Prostate Cancer

When your prostate cancer is diagnosed, your doctor will try to determine the *stage* of the cancer—whether it may have spread beyond the prostate. The progress of prostate cancers is fairly predictable. All begin as small lesions confined to the gland itself. In time, they spread first to other parts of the prostate, then to the seminal vesicles, then to the lymph nodes, and eventually to the bones in the spine, ribs, or pelvis, and beyond. The cancer's *clinical stage* is estimated by putting together pieces of evidence gathered from the DRE, the PSA, ultrasound, biopsy, and other tests. The more accurate *pathologic stage* is established when a pathologist examines the prostate gland after it is surgically removed.

There are two staging systems in widespread use, the *Whitmore-Jewett* and the *TNM*. In the United States, TNM (short for *T*umor, *N*odes, and *M*etastases) is used more than Whitmore-Jewett. For more information on these staging systems, see the Appendix.

Grading Prostate Cancer

In the mid-1970s, Dr. Donald Gleason developed a grading system to measure the appearance and arrangement of prostate cancer cells viewed under a microscope. How the cells look can tell a pathologist a lot about how aggressive the cancer is likely to be.

Healthy cells are well *differentiated*. It's easy to see the cell boundaries, where one cell stops and another begins. Malignant cells tend to be poorly differentiated; their shapes and boundaries are blurry, and the normal structure of the tissue is absent.

To assign a *grade* to prostate cancer cells, the pathologist looks at the two largest areas of cancer in the tissue sample and assigns *each* of them a number from 1 to 5. The higher the number, the more poorly differentiated are the cancer cells. The two numbers are then added together to make the *Gleason score.* The less differentiated (separate) and the more disorganized the cells appear, the more aggressive the cancer, and the higher the Gleason score.

Low Gleason scores of 2, 3, or 4 indicate well-differentiated cells with a more normal appearing structure. High scores from 8 to 10 mean that cells appear disorganized and are poorly differentiated, suggesting an aggressive, rapidly progressing cancer. Intermediate scores of 5, 6, and 7 indicate moderately differentiated cells.

> *Annual testing is so important that men should make it a calendar event, such as a birthday or Father's Day, or schedule testing each September, which is Prostate Cancer Awareness Month.*
> *—John Page, President, Us Too!*

Sometimes a pathologist examining biopsied prostate tissue will see abnormal cells that appear precancerous. This condition is called *prostatic intraepithelial neoplasia (PIN)* or *atypia.* PIN is classified in two groups: low and high grade. Low grade means the cells look normal. High grade mean the cells look abnormal. If you have a high-grade PIN, there is a 30 to 50 percent chance of having prostate cancer. Accordingly, your doctor will likely want to do a second biopsy.

To discover whether your prostate cancer is confined to the prostate, your doctor will take into consideration such factors as your PSA, clinical stage, and Gleason score. With this information at hand, doctors try to predict how your cancer might behave. Investigators at Johns Hopkins University, led by Dr. Allen Partin, took this approach one step further. By looking at thousands of prostates that had been removed and matching those to the patient's stage, Gleason grade, and PSA score, they were able to construct what are now called the *Partin Tables* to predict whether the cancer is confined to the prostate. You may wish to ask your doctor where your cancer ranks on the Partin Tables.

Other Tests and Studies

Your doctor may have access to a great variety of other procedures that offer even more specific information about your prostate cancer to help you choose the best treatment.

Bone Scan

If your PSA is greater than 10, your doctor might want to do a *bone scan* to determine whether a cancer has spread to the bones. Some doctors recommend it for all prostate cancer patients. A radioactive substance is inserted that is absorbed by your body in areas of rapid bone growth. Cancer cells in the bone stimulate new bone growth as a reaction and a special camera sees these areas as hot spots. However, other conditions, can show up as hot spots, including arthritis, healed bone fractures, and Paget's disease, a nonmalignant, metabolic bone disorder in which bone cells grow out of control.

ProstaScint

ProstaScint is a staging tool similar to a bone scan except that it finds hot spots in soft tissue rather than bones. ProstaScint is sometimes used with other imaging techniques, such as a CT scan of the pelvis, PET scans, and bone scans. The ProstaScint study is somewhat controversial, but is becoming more sensitive and selective for prostate cancer.

CT Scan

In a *computerized tomography scan (CT scan,* also called a *CAT scan*), a machine moves around your body to take a circular series of X-rays. A CT scan sees masses and other structures inside the body with much greater accuracy than standard X-rays; it painlessly and noninvasively reveals abnormalities in tissue and bone. This amazing tool can be helpful in many phases of diagnosis and treatment. Many doctors order a CT scan before starting radiation treatment to determine where and how much radiation is needed.

Magnetic Resonance Imaging

Like the CT scan, *magnetic resonance imaging (MRI)* presents a three-dimensional image, but uses magnetic waves rather than X-rays. Painless and noninvasive, it can identify bone abnormalities as cancerous or benign. The MRI produces a loud clanging sound, due to strong electromagnetic fields being switched off and on, that some patients find unpleasant. The test involves about 20-45 minutes of confinement in a tunnel-like structure. You can wear ear plugs or listen to music through head phones during the procedure. If you tend to be claustrophobic, your doctor might give you a light sedative.

I'm never offended if a patient asks for another opinion. Patients should look for a urologist who is board-certified, a member of the American Urological Association, and in good standing with the county medical society.
—Dr. Arthur Centeno
Urologist

A newer MRI scan, the spectroscopic MRI, has become more widely available and appears to be helpful in determining the extent of prostate cancer. This MRI is conducted in exactly the same way as the traditional prostate MRI, but in addition to examining soft tissue, it examines the levels of the chemicals choline and citrate in the prostate. It has been found that prostate cancer cells contain more choline and less citrate than normal tissues. MRI spectroscopy can actually measure the levels of these chemicals within the prostate gland and indicate which areas are suspicious for being cancerous.

PET Scan

For *positron emission tomography (PET)* scans, patients are injected with a sugar solution. Since tumor cells use glucose as an energy source, the sugar solution gravitates to cancerous tissue. As a result, PET scans can locate tumors and can tell how quickly they digest the sugar. The more rapid the digestion, the more likely it is that the cells are malignant. However, since prostate cancer cells are slow growing, they are less likely to light up on PET scans so PET scans are not used routinely in prostate cancer staging.

Laparoscopic Pelvic Lymphadenectomy

Laparoscopic pelvic lymphadenectomy (*LPLND*) is a less invasive alternative to open surgery for the evaluation of the pelvic lymph nodes in patients with prostate cancer. In this procedure, lymph nodes are removed from the pelvic area with the help of a laparascope, a viewing tube that contains a television camera. This scope is inserted into the lower abdomen through a small incision, making it possible for the surgeon to see the lymph nodes and surrounding tissues on a television camera. Using another tube-like instrument, which is inserted through another small incision, the surgeon removes the lymph nodes.

Once the lymph nodes are removed, they are sent to a pathology lab where they are checked for the presence of cancer.

Minilap

The *minilaparotomy* (*minilap*) *staging pelvic lymphadenectomy* involves a slightly larger incision than the lap procedure. If cancer is found in the lymph nodes, the incision is closed. Otherwise, the surgeon lengthens the incision and removes the prostate with a radical retropubic prostatectomy, which will be discussed in the next chapter.

After Diagnosis: Choosing a Treatment Plan

The diagnosing procedures described in this chapter give your doctor important information about the treatment method likely to be most effective. If you have been diagnosed with prostate cancer, you will be able to discuss treatment options with your doctor. As you may already know, the basic forms of treatment include surgery, radiation therapy, cryosurgery, hormone therapy, and chemotherapy. Treatment options are based on one's age, general health, and stage of the cancer at the time of diagnosis.

3

Surgery for Prostate Cancer

If you're considering surgery as one of your treatment options, you're in good company. Among men with early stage prostate cancer, surgery to remove the prostate, the seminal vesicles, and the pelvic lymph nodes is the most widely chosen treatment. Surgery may also offer the best chance for a cure. What does the word, "cure," mean in terms of a prostate cancer diagnosis? Nowadays, oncologists are careful about using the word; however, a man who has had his prostate gland surgically removed is generally considered cured if, five years later, he has no evidence of recurring cancer and his PSA level has not increased.

Are You a Candidate for Surgery?

You're most likely to benefit from surgery to remove the prostate if your cancer is confined to the prostate, you have fairly low-grade disease (Gleason score of 6 or less), your PSA level is 4 or less, you're in your early seventies or younger, and you're in good overall health with a normal life expectancy of at least ten more years.

There are, of course, exceptions to this profile. Your case is not exactly like anyone else's. Under certain circumstances, higher PSA levels and Gleason scores, cancer that may have spread to the seminal vesicles, and other unfavorable signs might not automatically exclude you from having radical surgery.

If you believe you might be a candidate for surgery and your doctor doesn't agree, find out why. If you're not satisfied with the answer, get a second opinion. Do your own research and talk to prostate cancer survivors. No reputable surgeon is going to perform a radical prostatectomy if he or she doesn't think it will be beneficial; however, you have the right to know why and to state your case.

Surgical Procedures

Radical Retropubic Prostatectomy

A *radical prostatectomy* is a major operation that usually takes two to four hours. It also requires two to four days in the hospital and several weeks' recovery at home. The term *radical,* in medicine, refers to a treatment meant to remove the source of an illness. You and your doctor may decide that the retropubic approach is best for you. *Retro* means behind, and *pubis* refers to the pubic area, the lower part of the abdomen.

In a *radical retropubic prostatectomy,* your prostate, seminal vesicles, and pelvic lymph nodes will be removed through an incision in your lower abdomen from just below the navel down to the pubic bone. The lymph nodes will be rushed to the lab and immediately frozen, and a pathologist will examine them for cancer. If there are malignant cells showing that cancer has escaped the prostate, the surgeon will probably not continue with the operation. Surgery is unlikely to remove all the cancer once it has spread, and other options will be better able to treat your cancer.

Some doctors, however, might choose to proceed with surgery to remove the prostate even if the pathologist finds cancer in the pelvic lymph nodes. The rationale here is that by removing as much cancer as possible, known as *debulking*, your body's immune system can do a better job of fighting the cancer that remains. Debulking is controversial, however, and most doctors are unwilling to put patients through the rigors of surgery if it is unlikely to remove all the cancer.

There's another reason for proceeding with the operation even if local metastases are found. Your doctor might be cautiously optimistic that a cure is possible—even when cancer has penetrated the prostate wall and may have spread to the seminal vesicles. Treatment in this case involves a combination of radical prostatectomy, radiation to the prostate bed, and *adjuvant* hormonal therapy.

Adjuvant therapy is treatment that follows the primary form of treatment.

Nerve-Sparing Prostatectomy

If cancer has not penetrated the prostate capsule, your surgeon may attempt a *nerve-sparing prostatectomy,* which preserves the *neurovascular bundles* on either side of

Radical Retropubic Prostatectomy

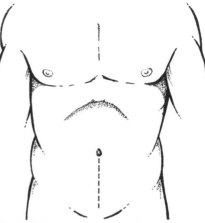

The incision for a radical retropubic prostatectomy is made in the abdomen, starting under the navel and extending to the pubic area.

your prostate. A few decades ago, these nerves were almost always cut during a radical prostatectomy, and patients had to live with permanent *impotence,* the inability to have an erection. These days surgeons can often preserve one or both neurovascular bundles. When the cancer appears to be located on only one side of your prostate, the surgeon might leave the nerves intact on the opposite side, if he or she is certain that no cancer cells will be left behind. It is not possible to remove only part of the prostate. Even if only one lobe appears cancerous, the doctor will remove the entire gland.

Radical Perineal Prostatectomy

Using the perineal approach, called *radical perineal prostatectomy*, doctors remove the prostate through an incision in the perineum rather than the abdomen. The perineal approach is less common than the retropubic for at least three reasons: it doesn't permit removal and dissection of the pelvic lymph nodes, it makes the nerve-sparing technique difficult, and the surgeon can't remove as much tissue. The retropubic incision (in the abdomen) places the prostate and surrounding organs and tissues in plain view and within comparatively easy access. Even though the perineal incision is used rather infrequently, it has advantages. The perineal incision is several inches shorter than the retropubic incision. Also, the perineal surgery is over in as little as an hour and a half, the recovery time is shorter as well, and less blood is lost than with the retropubic approach. Finally, perineal surgery might be better for obese patients since it provides easier access to the prostate gland.

Radical Perineal Prostatectomy

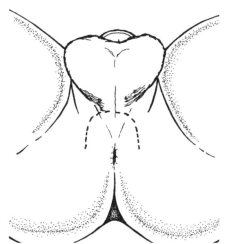

An incision for a perineal radical prostatectomy is made in the perineum, between the scrotum and the anus.

If you've decided on the perineal approach and your doctor wants to remove the pelvic lymph nodes for dissection, you'll have a separate procedure called a *lymphadenectomy*. Some surgeons use a traditional surgical approach through a small incision in the lower abdomen. Other surgeons remove the lymph nodes laparoscopically, a less invasive procedure.

Radical Laparoscopic Prostatectomy

Some surgeons in the United States are performing radical prostatectomies *laparoscopically*. For prostate removal, the surgeon makes a very small abdominal incision and inserts a small camera called an *endoscope* into the patient's abdomen. The endoscope projects images onto a video monitor, enabling the surgeon to see the prostate and surrounding area without the exposure and trauma of a full abdominal incision. In the most advanced laparoscopic technique, a robotic arm obeys the surgeon's spoken instructions to position the endoscope.

The advantages of the laparoscopic technique, should it eventually be proven as effective as open surgery, quickly come to mind: a smaller incision, comparatively little bleeding, much quicker recovery, and fewer complications. At this point the technique is so new that researchers don't know how successful it will be in the long run.

Before the Operation

Your doctor will schedule surgery at least four to six weeks after your needle biopsy or twelve weeks after surgery for benign prostatic hyperplasia. This waiting period will give the prostate and tissues surrounding it a chance to heal from the previous biopsy.

> *I had faith in my surgeon—he does 50 to 100 prostatectomies a year. With a Gleason score of 7, I felt surgery would provide me with the best opportunity to get the cancer totally out of my body.*
>
> *—Paul 67*

At the time the operation is scheduled, ask whether you should take your regular medications to the hospital when you check in for your surgery and tell your doctor about all prescription and over-the-counter drugs, food supplements, herbal products, and other remedies you are taking. The doctor will tell you when to stop taking some or all of these substances before the operation.

For example, seven to ten days before surgery, you'll probably have to stop taking products containing aspirin or ibuprofen, as well as vitamin E, fish oil, garlic tablets, and other potentially blood-thinning substances to prevent excessive bleeding during surgery. If another doctor has prescribed blood-thinning medication for you, let your surgeon know and check with the prescribing doctor before you stop taking it.

Some herbal supplements might interact with the anesthetic given during surgery. Your doctor may tell you to stop taking these products two weeks before your scheduled operation.

Be sure to let your doctor know if you have ever had blood clots. This information helps the anesthesiologist and the surgeon take extra precautions during surgery. To further reduce the risk of blood clots, your doctor will probably have you wear *pneumatic stockings,* which improve blood circulation by repeatedly inflating and deflating, during surgery and for a few days after.

To guard against infection, you'll start taking antibiotics before the operation and continue for a few days after. Your doctor will advise you to have an enema or take a laxative, or both, the night before surgery and will ask you not to eat for at least twelve hours before the operation begins. You might also be given a special antiseptic soap to shower with before surgery.

Receiving Anesthesia

You'll have a general anesthetic to put you to sleep and possibly an *epidural,* a drip into the epidural space near the base of the spine, to temporarily numb the lower part of your body. The epidural space contains nerves running from your spine to your lower body.

After an injection to numb the part of your back where the epidural will go in—similar to the Novocain shot you get at the dentist—an anesthesiologist will push a long, thin needle into the epidural space. Through the needle, a very narrow plastic tube called an epidural catheter will be inserted and the needle itself will be withdrawn. Epidural anesthesia prolongs recovery of bowel functions and sometimes requires an additional day or two in the hospital.

Undergoing Surgery

To perform a radical retropubic prostatectomy, the surgeon will begin by making the incision. If your doctor is using the retropubic approach, the veins that feed the area will be cut and cauterized to achieve what is called a *bloodless field.* In reality, you'll probably lose 350 to 500 cc of blood, less than the amount you'd donate to the Red Cross in one session.

As mentioned earlier, the surgeon will remove the pelvic lymph nodes, which a pathologist will examine immediately. This process, called a *staging pelvic lymphadenectomy,* is sometimes omitted if your Gleason score is lower than 8.

If the pathologist's report shows that your lymph nodes are clear of cancer and the operation continues, the surgeon will remove your prostate, the seminal vesicles, and if needed, one or both neurovascular bundles. In the lab, the pathologist will examine the prostate to determine the cancer's type, grade, extent, volume, and whether the surgical margins are clear. *Margins* refer to whether the cancer cells have spread outside the area of the incision. If cancer cells are found at the incision site, the margin it is called a *positive margin.* Whether the margin is positive is important because this increases the chance of a cancer recurrence, and your physician may offer you additional treatment. Results from this routine analysis will be available in a day or two.

> *I was 45 when I had a radical prostatectomy. I would follow the same path again. Two years post surgery, my follow-up tests have been negative. I still exercise daily, running and biking, as I did before the surgery.*
>
> —*Bill, 47*

The prostatic urethra—the part of the urethra surrounded by the prostate—will also be removed, and the surgeon will reattach the remaining urethra to the bladder neck with sutures. This new connection is called an *anastomosis,* a term worth remembering because you'll need to guard it well in the weeks to come. The surgeon will insert a Foley catheter through the penis to the bladder, anchoring it with a small balloon. While the catheter is in place, urine will bypass the anastomosis so it can heal properly. If the catheter is pulled loose or removed too soon, permanent incontinence—which is otherwise quite rare—could result.

In spite of measures to control bleeding during surgery, occasionally patients require blood transfusions. At the time your surgery is scheduled, ask your doctor if you should donate your own blood (*autologous donation*) for transfusions. Many surgeons feel that, because so few patients require transfusions, autologous donations are unnecessary, even wasteful.

After the Operation

You'll spend an hour or more in the recovery room, where you'll be monitored until the general anesthetic wears off. Very rarely, a patient will have an allergic reaction to the anesthetic used during surgery. Symptoms range from fever or a rash to swelling of the tongue and lips. If you notice any of these symptoms once you become conscious after surgery, be sure to report them without delay. A severe allergic reaction could be fatal.

You'll wake up to find several tubes projecting from your body. One or two of them will be drains placed during surgery to suction leakage from the anastomosis. They'll probably be removed before you leave the hospital. The Foley catheter, also placed during surgery, will drain urine from your bladder while the anastomosis heals. You'll have an IV in your arm for fluids and possibly for medication.

Your epidural tube may remain in place for pain relief medication. You'll probably receive a powerful nonnarcotic drug, better than narcotic pain relievers because it's unlikely to upset your stomach.

Your pain relief might come in the form of a *PCA pump*. PCA stands for *patient-controlled analgesia,* which means that you control the timing of your pain medication using a device with built-in safeguards against dosing too much or too often.

If you have to rely on hospital staff to administer pain medication, don't be timid. You've just had a major insult to the midsection and you have a right to be as comfortable as today's safe and effective medications can make you. The best advice: Don't wait for pain to become intense before seeking pain medication. Try to stay ahead of the pain.

Preventing Deep Venous Thrombosis

However capable your surgeon, preventing blood clots in the deep veins of the legs, called *deep venous thrombosis,* requires some effort on your part. It's your job to move about, since mobility keeps your blood circulating so clots don't have a chance to form.

Not only are these blood clots painful, they can be deadly. If a clot breaks off and travels through your body, it can move through your heart to a lung. A blood clot in the lung, a *pulmonary embolism,* can be fatal.

Cavernous Nerves

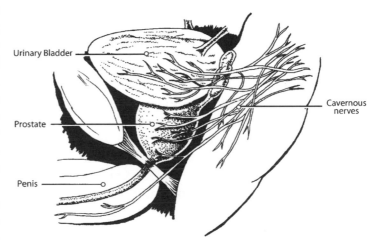

The cavernous nerves, which control erections, are attached to the prostate. These nerves can be easily damaged when the prostate is removed, affecting a man's ability to achieve an erection.

You'll be encouraged to walk for a few minutes every hour as soon as you're alert after surgery and for the entire time you're in the hospital. Once you're at home, you'll need to continue this regimen. No need to take a long stroll, which could tire you out. Frequent short walks will go a long way toward preventing blood clots. And don't sit for long on a firm surface with your legs hanging over the edge, which can restrict blood circulation in your legs. Elevate your legs as much as possible.

Recovery at Home

Within four weeks you should be able to return to your usual routine, unless that routine is particularly strenuous. Ask your doctor to recommend when you can resume heavy lifting, sports, and other vigorous activities. Remember that your body has just undergone a major shock and that your genitourinary system is fragile. Allowing your body to heal while exerting yourself no more than necessary for blood circulation will be your challenge in the days to come.

Caring for the Foley Catheter

You'll leave the hospital with the Foley catheter still in place and with two bags to collect the urine, a large bag to use at night and a smaller bag taped to your leg for daytime drainage. A tube connects the catheter to whichever drainage bag is in use.

Your doctor might suggest that you limit outings to an hour or so while you're using the Foley catheter. You probably won't feel much like going anywhere for a while anyway, but if you do leave the house, be sure the daytime drainage bag is placed lower than the catheter and is securely taped at all times.

The catheter is painless, but it requires some care and attention. Your doctor will give you detailed instructions to follow at home until your two-week checkup, when the catheter will mostly likely be removed. Until then, take showers rather than tub baths and don't get into a swimming pool, Jacuzzi, or sauna.

- Empty the drainage bags often to keep urine from backing up into your bladder—every three to four hours for the leg bag and every eight hours for the larger bag.

- Keep the bags, the tubing, and the connections clean.

- Stay squeaky clean yourself, washing the penis where the catheter exits and the rectal area a few times a day and after a bowel movement with soap and water.

- Don't pull on the catheter, and be sure there's enough slack in the tube so that you won't pull it out accidentally when turning over in your sleep, for example.

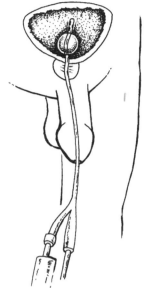

A Foley catheter is used to drain urine from the bladder when normal urination is disrupted. The catheter is threaded through the urinary duct (urethra) and into the bladder.

Managing Incontinence

Once your catheter is removed you'll notice some urine leakage. Though it's almost certainly a temporary inconvenience, it can still cause you great embarrassment.

Don't drink more than two quarts of water a day for a while and limit caffeine and alcohol to avoid undue stress on the anastomosis, the new connection between the urethra and the bladder neck. Ask your doctor when the anastomosis is likely to be fully healed.

The return of continence is gradual. Meanwhile, your doctor can recommend incontinence products, pads or special underwear, you can use to stay comfortable and avoid embarrassment. To help regain control of the urinary sphincter, the muscle that controls the release of urine from your bladder, do *Kegel exercises,* which involve tightening the sphincter to stop the flow of urine. You can practice these when you urinate, but ask your doctor how to do them properly and how often.

Coping with Impotence

Impotence, or erectile dysfunction, does *not* mean that your sex life is over or that it can't be just as exciting and pleasurable as before the operation. If you're in your forties or fifties, you'll most likely regain your ability to have an erection, especially if your surgeon used the nerve-sparing technique, but it will take time. Your doctor can tell you what to expect, and a prostate cancer support group can offer valuable reassurance.

> *I had surgery five years ago and I feel great. I was 39 years old at the time of my diagnosis. I tell every guy I know to insist on an annual DRE and PSA.*
> *—Todd, 44*

Your doctor might prescribe Viagra or one of the newer drugs, Levitra or Cialis, now available for erectile dysfunction. Or he or she may recommend a vacuum device a month or six weeks after surgery to improve circulation in the penis. Two to four months after surgery, after you've been on one of these drugs for a while, your doctor may "prescribe" sexual activity. If you are still impotent at that time, the doctor may begin penile injection therapy. Chapter 8 contains more information about ways to cope with impotence.

Keeping Bowels Regular

The part of the rectum adjacent to the prostate will be fragile, and you'll need to give it time to heal. It may be a few days after surgery before you have a bowel movement, which should be painless if you take milk of magnesia or use stool softeners, according to your doctor's instructions. Avoid straining, which could injure the rectum.

For three months or so after your operation, do not have an enema or take your temperature rectally. Try to have a bowel movement every day, continuing to take stool softeners and a laxative if necessary, according to your doctor's instructions. Drinking two quarts of water every day and eating fiber can keep you from getting constipated.

Guarding Against Infection

Most of the healing of your incision takes place within six weeks after surgery, but it will continue to heal for up to a year. Infections are very uncommon. If your incision or the IV site on your arm is extremely tender or puffy, tell your doctor right away. Antibiotic medication will usually take care of the problem.

Returning to Normal Activities

Follow your doctor's instructions about what you can do and when. The first week you'll want to take it easy. Catch up on television programs, lay in a supply of good books or crossword puzzles, rest, and drink plenty of fluids. Once you're home, you can probably return to your normal diet as long as it doesn't make you constipated. This would be a good time, however, to change your eating habits if your normal diet is high in animal fat and low in fiber.

The second week you'll feel much better. You might be bored and want to get out and do things. Ask your doctor how much activity is *too* much. Many doctors recommend staying off your feet as much as possible or doing nothing more strenuous than a short walk. You might want to take someone with you on your first stroll to the end of the block, in case you get there and find you're too worn out to get home.

During that second week your bladder may start to rebel against the catheter. You'll experience bladder spasms, annoying cramps that come and go, and probably some urine leakage around the catheter.

My prostate cancer was diagnosed when I was 58. My family doctor sent me to a urologist and within six weeks I had a radical prostatectomy. Since then I've been presented with four grandchildren I would have never known without the right diagnosis and treatment.

—Luis, 70

The best remedy is rest and adequate fluids. Take four to six short walks each day to keep your blood moving without exhausting yourself.

You should be able to return to work after three or four weeks if you have a desk job. Stay home a few weeks longer if your job requires heavy lifting or being on your feet a lot.

To give your sutures a chance to heal, don't lift anything over ten pounds for the first six weeks. Don't drive for at least four weeks, as much for others' safety as for your own. Your reaction time will be slower than before and you might have trouble stopping quickly in an emergency. Wait at least six weeks after surgery to play golf or tennis, bowl, lift weights, or ride a bicycle.

Postsurgical Doctor Visits

You'll see your doctor a week to ten days after surgery, and your incision will be checked. Your sutures will likely be removed at this time. Two weeks after surgery, your doctor will likely remove the Foley catheter. When the catheter is first removed, you might have temporary *stress urinary incontinence*—urine leakage when you sneeze, for example, or stand up after sitting. Kegel exercises can help.

Two to six weeks after surgery, you'll probably meet with your doctor to go over your pathology report and plan any long-term follow-up care. As often as every three months for the first year and at least once a year thereafter, you will have follow-up visits with your doctor. This may be more than one doctor; for example, if you had surgery and then have radiation therapy, you could schedule appointments with both doctors on the same day.

During your postsurgical visits your doctor will likely perform a DRE and a PSA blood test. The doctor will be checking for evidence of any recurrence as well as any complications from treatment. Your doctor will ask you about any urinary symptoms such as frequent urination, slow stream, leakage of urine, and burning sensations when urinating. You'll also likely be asked about any bowel symptoms such as diarrhea and rectal blood or mucus.

Risks, Complications, and Side Effects

As you read about risks and possible complications of prostate surgery, please keep in mind that the percentages are drawn from the entire prostate cancer population. These risks, most of which are low to begin with, are even less likely in the hands of a skilled and experienced surgeon.

Some men are more frightened about risks and side effects than they are about the cancer itself. If you are one of these men, please take a minute to consider the statistics on risks.

Risks during or soon after a radical prostatectomy:

- The risk of death is less than one-half of 1 percent.
- The risk of life-threatening complications is lower than 1 percent.
- The risk of severe incontinence is about 2 –3 percent .
- The risk of impotence is about 30 percent for men in their forties and rises with age to about 80 percent for men in their seventies. Impotence refers only to the ability to have an erection. It does not affect physical sensation or arousal or the ability to have an orgasm. Furthermore, there are several effective remedies for impotence, such as medications and surgical implants.
- The risk of *urethral stricture* is lower than 10 percent. This narrowing of the urethra is caused by scar tissue that forms after surgery. It can be "stretched" by a urologist in an outpatient procedure.
- The risk of deep venous thrombosis—blood clots in the deep veins of the legs—is about 10 percent, much lower with

routine preventive measures such as pneumatic stockings and blood-thinning medication.

- The most common side effect of the epidural is itching. Other epidural side effects, breathing difficulty and infection, are extremely rare.
- Highly unusual after prostatectomy are urinary tract infections, stomach ulcers, pneumonia, and allergic reactions to medication.
- The risk of bowel injury is about one-half of 1 percent. Any such injury can likely be repaired during your operation.

As you can see, the odds are overwhelmingly in your favor, especially if you're younger than 70.

When to Call the Doctor

Call your doctor, call 911, or go to a hospital emergency room immediately if you have nausea, vomiting, difficulty breathing, fever over 100°F, chills, a rash, *any* swelling or redness, or unusual pain, especially in your legs or chest; if you think your catheter is blocked; or if you cough up blood. Some of these symptoms could indicate blood clots, which can be fatal. Treatment with anticoagulant (anticlotting) medication is usually effective when started immediately. If you have these symptoms in the middle of the night, don't wait till morning to report them.

4

Radiation Therapy

Radiation therapy has come a long way since 1895 when the X-ray was discovered, and since the early part of the twentieth century when Marie Curie published her groundbreaking "Theory of Radioactivity." In your father's or grandfather's day, radiation treatments were less effective than they are now and carried a greater chance of injuring healthy tissue.

Today you have the benefit of higher energy radiation beams and of beam-shaping devices that target tumors more precisely. Sophisticated imaging studies such as MRI, CT, and PET scans produce multidimensional pictures and allow multidimensional planning and guidance before and during your radiation treatments. Powerful computers record information about your treatments and calculate radiation dosages high enough to be effective, but with minimal damage to surrounding healthy cells.

Like surgery, radiation is an aggressive prostate cancer treatment. In fact, radiation therapy is used in more than half of all cancer cases in the United States. If you're a good candidate for radiation, you might be more comfortable with the risks and possible side effects than you are with those of surgery.

Studies indicate that radiation is as effective as surgery for seven to fifteen years; however, results after that point are significantly better for surgery. Accordingly, radical prostatectomy is still the preferred curative therapy for younger men, those who could reasonably expect to live for another ten years or more.

It can be tricky, however, to compare the various forms of treatment for at least two reasons. First, treatment technologies are advancing so quickly there hasn't been time for long-term studies to produce solid data on results. Second, the studies that do exist often aren't standardized, measuring different time periods, risk groups, and therapy combinations. Balancing the results can be like comparing apples to oranges. Still, there's solid evidence that men who choose radiation can live for many years after treatment, often without lasting incontinence, impotence, or other troublesome side effects.

Before you decide on a course of radiation therapy for your prostate cancer, talk to others who have had radiation therapy. Discuss your concerns with your doctor, and consider a second opinion from a physician who does not specialize in radiation therapy. You might decide that radiation is indeed the best option for you, but you'll feel better about your decision if you've explored the alternatives.

How Radiation Works

Radiation is effective in killing fast-growing cells. Cancer cells are fast growing. Radiation treatment uses high-energy particles or waves to damage the genetic material in the cancer cells that controls their division and growth.

The goal of radiation therapy is to kill cancer cells while sparing nearby healthy cells. Though some healthy tissue damage is unavoidable, normal cells are better able to repair the damage than cancer cells.

There are two types of radiation therapy, brachytherapy and external beam radiation therapy. Radiation therapy is administered by a doctor known as a *radiation oncologist.*

Hormone Treatment Before Radiation

It is common for prostate cancer patients being treated with radiation to have hormonal therapy for several months before radiation begins. Such therapy given before the primary treatment begins is called neoadjuvant therapy. If your prostate gland is enlarged, your doctor will probably recommend this course of treatment. Neoadjuvant hormonal therapy may also be recommended if your PSA is 10 or higher or your Gleason score is 6 or higher, either of which may place you at medium to high risk for recurrence.

Hormonal therapy shrinks prostate tissues, both normal and cancerous, by depriving them of testosterone, which they must have to grow and reproduce. The smaller the tumor, the more precisely radiation can be targeted and the less likely the destruction of normal cells.

Brachytherapy

One of the two basic types of radiation treatment, *brachytherapy* (BRACK-ee-therapy), also called *seed implantation*, involves the placement of tiny radioactive seeds or pellets directly into the prostate gland. The prefix *brachy-* comes from a Greek word for "short" or "nearby"; in this case, it refers to the fact that the seeds are close to the cancerous tissue. You may also come across the term *interstitial brachytherapy.* Interstitial means "within the tissues," in this case, within the prostate gland.

What's most important? Find a doctor who treats lots of men with prostate cancer. My husband, 73, is alive because he has a smart, experienced urologist who wanted my husband to understand the choice he was making. He had radiation and has been cancer free for five years.
—Edie, wife of a survivor

Permanent Seed Implantation

There are two types of brachytherapy. The first and most commonly used is the *permanent seed implant (PSI).* As the name implies, the implanted seeds are not removed. Over the ensuing days, weeks, and months, the seeds release radiation that destroys nearby cancer cells. After a period of months, the radioactivity decays.

Temporary Seed Implantation

The second type of brachytherapy is *temporary seed implantation*, also called *high-dose-rate* (*HDR*) brachytherapy. The seed is a single highly radioactive pellet that is not left in the body. This type of brachytherapy can deliver more intense radiation than permanent seeds, and may be more advantageous to men in a higher risk category. The higher the radiation dose, the better the job it does of destroying cancer cells; but a dose that is too high can inflict excessive damage on healthy tissue and create permanent, unacceptable side effects, including severe bowel and urinary problems.

HDR has several advantages over permanent seeds. The higher dose radiation can be more powerful against cancer. Also, the distribution of the radiation dose near the urethra can be optimized without increased risk of injury to the urethra. However, most of the data on long-term effectiveness of brachytherapy comes from permanent seed implants. Accordingly, most radiation oncologists still prefer permanent seed implantation.

Before Brachytherapy

Preparing for brachytherapy is similar in many ways to preparing for radical prostatectomy. Usually, you'll have to wait eight to twelve weeks after you begin hormonal therapy to give the prostate a chance to shrink. You'll also start taking antibiotics shortly before to prevent infection. As with surgery, you'll be told when to stop taking blood-thinning medications and other drugs or supplements that might make your treatment more difficult or risky. Some doctors tell their radiation therapy patients to stop taking antioxidant supplements (vitamins C, E, and selenium), which may interfere with cancer cell destruction.

With both permanent and temporary brachytherapy, seed placement will be planned and dosages calculated ahead of time with X-rays, CT scans, ultrasound, PET scans, or other imaging techniques. Two to six weeks before seed implantation, you will also have what is called a *planning study* performed on an outpatient basis. During this study, the doctor will insert an ultrasound probe through the rectum; an enema the night before will provide a clear field of view. The probe will project images onto a television monitor. The computer software has a superimposed grid, to help the doctor determine where to implant the radioactive seeds.

Your doctor might also schedule an electro-cardiogram (EKG), blood tests, and a chest X-ray. These tests help your doctor decide what kind of anesthetic to use. You may also have a staging pelvic lymphadenectomy, a brief operation to sample the pelvic lymph nodes and examine them for cancer. If the procedure finds that cancer has spread, your doctor will probably recommend a treatment such as hormonal therapy.

I had 32 radiation treatments. I am now two years down the road. My PSA is at 0.05, and my Zoladex injections are finished. The best thing is that I still have a positive outlook on life. I am lucky I received a diagnosis early.

—John, 53

Your doctor may prescribe a blood thinner if you have a history of blood clots, but this will be done only if the doctor determines it will not cause excessive bleeding. Just prior to your brachytherapy treatment, your doctor might also prescribe a steroid to prevent swelling from the procedure. You will probably be instructed to have an enema the night before your radiation treatment and to eat nothing after midnight.

Delivery of Brachytherapy

The procedure to insert permanent radioactive seeds takes about an hour. You'll probably check in to the hospital the day of the

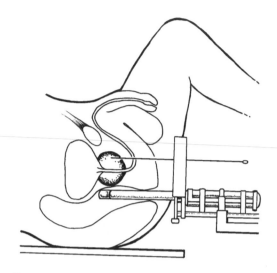

During a seed implant, an ultrasound probe, inserted in the rectum, helps the physician guide needle-like instruments into the prostate, where the radioactive seeds are delivered.

procedure, which will be done under general anesthetic or local anesthetic with sedation. Many patients receive an epidural anesthetic to numb them from the waist down and possibly a sedative to make them relaxed. You may have intravenous antibiotics during the treatment.

In years past, nothing but eyesight and instinct guided doctors in seed placement. Today, doctors use high-tech imaging equipment and computer software to localize the prostate, determine where to place the seeds, and calculate dosages. To begin the implantation, the doctor will once again insert an ultrasound probe into the rectum. The ultrasound probe projects images onto a TV monitor to ensure precise seed placement. A perineal template, attached to the probe, has a grid with tiny holes in it. This grid is sutured to the perineum. Long, thin needles are then used to guide catheters through the template holes and into the prostate gland, where the radioactive seeds are implanted. Approximately 50 to 100 seeds are inserted. Each seed is about the size of a grain of rice. Rows of seeds are deposited uniformly throughout the prostate so that the radiation can cover the entire gland.

The procedure to insert temporary seeds is similar to that of implanting permanent seeds. The main difference, of course, is that the temporary seeds are not left in the prostate. For a temporary seed implant, between 20 and 49 narrow plastic catheters are guided into the prostate. The number of catheters inserted depends on the size of the prostate gland, with a larger gland requiring more catheters to treat a larger volume of tissue. These catheters remain in place for 24 to 36 hours, and you will probably have two or three treatments during this time. During the treatment, one radioactive seed travels in and out of each catheter. A computer program "instructs" the seed where and how long to dwell in any position in the catheters. The entire treatment takes only a day or two.

After Brachytherapy

After either form of brachytherapy, you'll spend an hour or more in the recovery room until the general anesthetic wears off. Then, you'll be able to go home that day or the next. You'll be given pain medication, and the Foley catheter will probably be removed if you have had a permanent seed implant. You may be given oral antibiotics to take for several days. You'll be able to resume most of your activities right away, including going back to work.

After permanent seed implantation, you should wait four to six weeks before having sex, and use a condom for as long as your doctor recommends. Some men who have had permanent implants are concerned that they might be "radioactive." It's very unlikely that the radiation could harm others you come into contact with. To be on the safe side, however, avoid close contact with babies, small children, and pregnant women for several weeks after

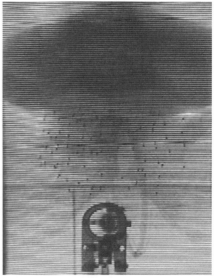

This X-ray was taken after brachytherapy, in which several dozen radioactive seeds were implanted in the prostate gland.

treatment. As an additional precaution, underwear that is lined with lead can be worn for two months following the procedure.

Follow-Up Visits to Your Doctor

After brachytherapy, you'll need to see your radiation oncologist every three to six months for a DRE and a PSA blood test. As in all follow-up visits, doctors are being vigilant, watching for any signs of cancer recurrence or complications from treatment.

If you've had permanent seed implants, your doctor will probably do a CT scan a few days to a month after treatment. Your doctor will check for any cold spots, areas that the seeds are not reaching with radiation. If a cold spot is discovered, the doctor may compensate with external beam radiation as long as the radiation dose to the rectum does not exceed its tolerance. Or the doctor may simply observe you. The five-year survival rate does not seem to be adversely affected by a cold spot. Most centers do not re-implant additional seeds.

External Beam Radiation Therapy

The second basic type of radiation therapy is *external beam radiation*, also called *EBRT* or *XRT*. This form of treatment uses radiation beams from outside the body to destroy cancers. Treatments typically are given five days a week, Monday through Friday, over a seven- to eight-week period. Weekend breaks are important, giving normal cells a chance to repair themselves.

For well-chosen radiation candidates, EBRT can be as effective and as safe as seed implantation. In part, that's because newer techniques allow much greater precision than conventional EBRT, which uses lead blocks to keep radiation from damaging the rectum, bladder, urethra, and other structures.

More modern methods, by contrast, make it possible to *conform* the radiation beams precisely to the target. This is much like a high-powered garden hose trigger can be adjusted to deliver a strong, narrow blast rather than a diffuse spray. *Conformal EBRT* does a better job of protecting bone marrow where blood cells are formed, as well as the rectum, bladder, and urethra, and is now standard treatment at most centers.

External Beam Radiation

Before External Beam Radiation

Prior to starting treatments, you will have a simulation, or planning session, in which the doctor outlines the radiation target and a physicist develops a radiation treatment plan. The simulation process takes about 20 minutes. You'll lie on a simulation couch—a narrow, rectangular table—and after you're injected with iodine contrast material, a CT scan will identify your prostate and surrounding tissues. The area to be treated will literally be drawn on your body with a marker, and tiny permanent ink tattoos will be placed in the corners and/or center of the area.

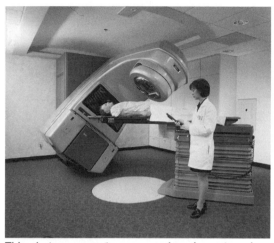

This photo represents a man undergoing external beam radiation therapy. Photo courtesy Varian Medical Systems of Palo Alto, California.

It's important that you remain absolutely still during your treatments. To keep your body still, an *immobilization device* will be prepared. The device might be a bag filled with a chemical that turns to Styrofoam and conforms to your shape when you lie on it. Or you might lie on a bag filled with Styrofoam pellets while technologists form a mold by suctioning out the air with a machine similar to a vacuum cleaner.

To be sure you're completely familiarized with the treatment process, you'll have a dry run before your first treatment.

Delivery of External Beam Radiation

When it's time for your treatment, you'll be asked to empty your bladder, then you'll undress from the waist down and cover yourself with a gown and a towel as you lie down on a table. Radiation therapy technologists may spend ten minutes or more arranging your body in the correct position as directed by the tattoos to make sure the radiation is focused precisely on the target. In fact, some radiation therapy centers use *BAT,* which stands for *B-mode acquisition and targeting.* This is a special ultrasound-based locating device system, designed to maximize the precision of external beam radiation. The prostate gland can change position, according to the fullness of the bladder and rectum. The B-mode system indicates whether the technologist needs to make subtle shifts in the treatment table position, based on tumor location, pinpointed by ultrasound.

> *Most external beam radiation therapy is preceded by hormonal therapy to downsize the prostate cancer so that the radiation has less effect on tissues of the bladder, rectum, and normal surrounding tissues.*
> *—Dr. Carol Kornmehl*
> *Radiation Oncologist*

Unlike brachytherapy, EBRT requires no incision or anesthesia. You'll simply lie still while radiation beams are directed at your prostate and the surrounding area.

The treatments themselves last five minutes or less. You won't feel anything on your skin, and all you'll hear is the whir of the EBRT machine, called a *linear accelerator.* It is a high-energy X-ray treatment unit that moves around your body sending precisely calculated doses of radiation to the tumor.

Intensity-modulated radiation therapy (IMRT) is even more sophisticated than conformal EBRT. In IMRT, multiple "beamlets" coming from many directions combine to create one conformal radiation beam. Each IMRT treatment takes about twenty minutes.

Other new variations of EBRT may differ from the conventional approach according to what kinds of radiation particles are used. Proton and neutron beam therapies are promising, but not yet widely available.

As you enter the latter weeks of treatment, you might feel tired, but you'll regain your normal energy shortly after the treatment ends. You should not experience pain; external beam therapy does not require pain medications.

After External Beam Radiation

Since external beam radiation treatment does not require any incisions, the recovery time is shorter than from brachytherapy. Some fatigue is likely, since your body will have experienced some major insults. However, many doctors believe that the fatigue associated with radiation is as much a result of psychological stress and sleep deprivation from nighttime urination and hormone-induced hot flashes than it is of the radiation itself.

Once your treatment is completed, your doctor will ask you to schedule follow-up visits every three to six months. As with other follow-ups, you will have blood drawn for PSA testing and DRE.

Are You a Candidate for Radiation Therapy?

Radiation treatment is best suited to patients whose cancer is confined to the prostate. It can be a good alternative to radical prostatectomy for older men or for those who are not robust enough to undergo invasive surgery.

Men with large tumors or enlarged prostate glands are not the best candidates for radiation, though pretreatment with hormone therapy may shrink the tissues enough to make radiation an option. EBRT is a better option than brachytherapy if you've had a TURP (transurethral resection of the prostate) procedure for benign prostatic hyperplasia. Why? Because if the prostate gland has been "hollowed out" with a TURP procedure, there is usually not enough tissue to anchor the radioactive seeds. And because external beam therapy can be directed to the prostate, seminal vesicles, and pelvic lymph nodes, it obviously can cover a larger area than seed implantation, which is usually restricted to the prostate itself.

For EBRT, a major consideration is whether you have a treatment center near you, especially one that offers the newer 3D conformal or IMRT. If not, you're looking at the time and expense involved in commuting to a regional center and/or finding lodging for two months or so. The typical EBRT schedule—Monday through Friday treatments for at least six weeks—is a key part of the treatment's effectiveness. You can't, for example, take a few weeks off in the middle.

Brachytherapy alone is usually recommended for those patients who are at low risk for recurrence. Patients with PSAs over 10, Gleason scores of 7 or above, and extensive cancers in both sides of the gland will usually be offered a combination of brachytherapy and EBRT.

Risks, Complications, and Side Effects

Most men tolerate radiation therapy well. Lasting side effects are uncommon. The risk of death or life-threatening complications is very low with any form of radiation therapy. Still, it is important to be aware of potential side effects. The side effects listed here may occur after either brachytherapy or external beam radiation therapy, but are more common after external beam radiation.

Whatever form of radiation you've been treated with, report all uncomfortable or alarming symptoms to your doctor, who can offer remedies ranging from diet and medication to brief outpatient surgery.

Recurrence or Metastases

The greatest complication from radiation therapy is local recurrence or metastases after seven to ten years. Even radiation's strongest advocates say that radical surgery is the best treatment for healthy men in their sixties or younger—men who could reasonably expect to live another ten years or longer if their prostate cancer is cured.

Incontinence and Impotence

Severe incontinence occurs in fewer than 2 percent of men treated with radiation. Impotence varies greatly immediately after radiation, from 25 to 50 percent among men age 60 or younger. Impotence and incontinence occasionally worsen in the months and years after treatment because irradiated healthy cells may lose the ability to repair themselves. As is the case after surgery, there are a number of effective treatments.

Common Short-Term Complications

For brachytherapy patients, short-term genital problems are common after radiation. Symptoms can include tenderness where brachytherapy needles were inserted, sore testicles or penis, and pain during ejaculation.

For both brachytherapy and ERBT patients, other side effects may include urine leakage (temporary incontinence), frequent need to urinate, difficulty urinating, and stinging or burning during urination or bowel movements. You might see blood in your urine, feces, or semen. These problems will probably go away on their own within a few weeks after treatment, but be sure to mention them to your doctor.

If urinary retention is acute, you'll feel bladder pressure but won't be able to urinate. Up to 15 percent of men require a Foley catheter for four to six weeks after radiation.

Men who have had ERBT may experience diarrhea as a side effect.

Urethral Stricture

With both forms of radiation treatment, there is a slight risk of *urethral stricture,* a shrinking of the urethra caused by scar tissue. A physician can "stretch" it back to size in an outpatient procedure.

Rectal Injury

Both forms of radiation treatment carry a risk of injury to the rectum. The first sign of such injury is often blood or mucus in the stool. Usually such injury can be repaired with laser surgery or cortisone-containing suppositories or enemas. If damage is severe, which is rare, major surgery may be necessary.

Infection or Expelled Seeds

Occasionally the prostate can become infected shortly after permanent or temporary seed implantation, requiring treatment with antibiotics. Rarely, seeds work their way out of the body through urine or semen (one of the reasons it's important to use a condom for a few months). If this happens, do not touch the seeds. Pick them up with rubber or vinyl gloves, wrap them securely in several layers of newspaper, and discard the gloves and the seeds in an outdoor trash container with a tight-fitting lid. The amount of radiation emitted is unlikely to be harmful, but you want to be sure that children or animals do not come in contact with them.

If you should expel a seed into the toilet, simply flush it. Retrieving it would likely mean greater exposure to radiation. Flushing one seed will not harm the environment.

PSA Bump

More than a third of men treated with brachytherapy experience a PSA bump eight to ten months after radiation. This temporary PSA elevation is almost always due to prostatitis, or prostate inflammation, rather than recurrent prostate cancer.

Other Types of Radiation Treatments

Combination Treatments

Your doctor might recommend EBRT or brachytherapy alone or in combination, though brachytherapy is usually combined with EBRT, hormone therapy, or both. EBRT can boost the radiation dosage delivered by permanently implanted seeds. Your doctor may recommend supplementing brachytherapy with EBRT if there's a high risk of cancer outside the prostate, but still confined to the seminal vesicles and pelvic lymph nodes.

Because radiation therapy is not ideal for large tumors, many doctors prefer to shrink bulky prostate cancer tumors and the prostate itself with hormone therapy before beginning a course of radiation treatment. Hormone therapy accomplishes this shrinkage by depriving the prostate cells, cancerous and normal cells alike, of the testosterone they depend on to survive and grow.

Five years ago, I had 37 radiation treatments. I traveled by van 70 miles a day with other cancer patients to a treatment center. My treatment went well and I enjoyed meeting the other people.

—Gene, 72

Radiation and Salvage Therapy

When a treatment fails, either because of local (pelvic area) recurrence or distant metastases, doctors often recommend *salvage therapy*. Salvage treatments may be given in the hope that a cure is still possible, especially if the recurrence is confined to the prostate, which is probable with a Gleason score of 7 or lower. Otherwise, salvage treatments can prolong life by controlling if not eliminating the cancer.

Every form of prostate cancer treatment, no matter how skillfully applied, takes its toll on the body, especially on the rectum, urethra, bladder, nerves, and blood vessels in the pelvic region. For that reason, only certain salvage therapies can be tried after other treatments have failed.

It's very unlikely, for example, that your doctor would recommend a radical prostatectomy after radiation treatments failed to eliminate the cancer from your body. For one thing, removing the prostate at that point would probably not remove all the cancer. Moreover, the odds of severe incontinence and impotence are much greater than with surgery or radiation alone.

On the other hand, EBRT is a possible salvage therapy if prostate cancer recurs locally after prostatectomy. EBRT can also be used for recurrence after brachytherapy, although it carries an increased risk of irritation or damage to both the urethra and the rectum.

Seed implantation is seldom used as salvage therapy. It is effective only if cancer is confined to the prostate. As mentioned earlier, if the prostate has been removed (or hollowed out with TURP to treat benign prostatic hyperplasia), there's often no good way to anchor the seeds.

Cryosurgery may be used for salvage therapy in some patients when radiation therapy fails. More information on this option is provided in the next chapter.

Long-term side effects are almost always increased by salvage therapy. There are effective remedies for these side effects, however, and most men are willing to take the risk if there's a chance for a cure or significant remission of their cancer.

Palliative Radiation

In cases of advanced prostate cancer, radiation can lessen pain and ease other symptoms. Patients with diffuse (widespread) bone pain can have injections of Metastron (strontium-89 chloride) or another radio-active isotope that seeks out bone metastases. Local EBRT treatments, sometimes called *spot radiation*, are effective for less diffuse metastases.

When to Call the Doctor

Call the doctor right away if you are unable to urinate. This is probably not a medical emergency, but it does require prompt treatment. Also call your doctor if you have any blood or excessive mucus in your stool, or severe pain.

Call your doctor, call 911, or go to a hospital emergency room *immediately* if you have symptoms of severe inflammation or infection—nausea, vomiting, fever of 100°F, or chills. Though blood clots are even less likely than after surgery, there's a very small chance of deep venous thrombosis—blood clots that could travel from the legs to the lungs—after seed implantation. Symptoms include pain or swelling in the legs, trouble breathing, or chest pain.

5

Prostate Cryoablation

You may not be as familiar with cryoablation as you are with other cancer treatments such as surgery, radiation, and chemotherapy. *Cryoablation*—"destruction by freezing"—is perhaps best known for its role in skin cancer treatment. The same principle is at work when cryoablation is used to destroy internal cancers such as those of the prostate. In these procedures, doctors apply supercooled instruments directly to cancerous tissue, killing the cancer but sparing surrounding healthy tissues from damage.

Cryoablation kills cancer cells in several ways: from ice forming within the cells, from the swelling and shrinking as cells freeze and then thaw, and from the loss of blood supply to the cells. Your body's white blood cells then take care of cleaning up the dead tissues.

Cryoablation, also called *cryotherapy* or *cryosurgery,* is fairly new as a prostate cancer treatment. It has been found effective both as a primary prostate cancer treatment and as salvage therapy.

History of Cyroablation

Cryoablation has been used since the 1960s to remove skin tumors and precancerous moles. As a treatment for prostate cancer, cryoablation met with limited success in the mid-1970s when University of Iowa surgeons placed *cryoprobes*, instruments that achieve extremely low temperatures, directly on prostate tumors during open surgery.

However, technology did not yet exist to allow doctors to see the extent of the freezing.

Interest was revived in the early 1990s after cryoablation, now aided by ultrasound imaging to guide placement of cryoprobes, was found to be successful in treating liver cancer. By 1993, published research confirmed prostate cancer treatment success using cryoablation. In 2002, the American Urological Association deemed cryoablation of the prostate a "standard" rather than "investigational" procedure. Today, some three hundred doctors perform cryoablation of the prostate.

Undergoing Cryoablation

The procedure involves two to three hours under general anesthetic. No major incision is required. The procedure is similar to brachytherapy, except that cryoprobes rather than radiation-loaded needles are placed through the skin of the perineum. The probes are about the size of small knitting needles. After insertion, the cryoprobe tips are supercooled with argon gas. Ultrasound monitoring allows the surgeon to apply the cryoprobes very accurately. Meanwhile, a urethral warming catheter circulates warm water through the urethra to protect it from the cold temperatures.

I had cryosurgery five years ago. I was in the hospital overnight and came home the next morning. Since then, my PSA has stayed around 0.2 to 0.4. I also have had follow-up biopsies and annual exams. All tests have been negative for cancer, so I am considered cured.

—Bill, 69

The surgeon can see the frozen tissues on the ultrasound monitor and can tailor the treatment to the tumor's shape and location. Probes are placed at sites toward the front, middle, and back of the prostate, and are activated in that order so that the surgeon can see the freezing process. After the cancerous tissues are frozen and thawed two or three times, the surgeon removes the cryoprobes and inserts a Foley catheter to drain the urine, since prostate swelling will obstruct the urethra for a time. The catheter will remain in place from a few days to as long as three weeks, depending on the extent of freezing. Note that some physicians prefer to use a suprapubic tube rather than a Foley catheter; the suprapubic tube enters the bladder through an incision in the lower abdomen, whereas the Foley enters through the penis.

Temperature monitoring with special probes placed in critical areas of the prostate is essential to the safety and success of your cryosurgery. The temperature of the prostate tumor must plunge to 40 degrees below zero or lower during two or three different freezes to destroy the cancer cells.

The best way to kill cancer with cryoablation is to freeze it rapidly and thaw it slowly. Waiting for the gland to thaw takes time, so some doctors use a thawing mode on the cryoprobes to speed up the process. This may be more convenient for the surgeon but less effective for the patient. Discuss this with your doctor and don't be reluctant to state your preference for the slower thawing method, which might mean the difference between eradicating cancer cells and temporarily stunning them.

To avoid injury to the rectum from freezing, many doctors are using a simple, newer technique that involves injecting a saline solution into the space between the rectum and the prostate. This separates these organs enough to keep the rectum from freezing, while allowing adequate freezing of the prostate cancer. With this technique, local cancer recurrence rates after cryosurgery fall to less than 5 percent.

After the Procedure

Cryoablation of the prostate requires an overnight stay in the hospital. On the evening after your treatment, you'll probably be able to eat a light meal and walk around a bit.

Plan to relax for the first five days at home, doing nothing more strenuous than going for brief walks. To relieve swelling around the scrotum and perineum, apply ice packs as directed by your doctor. Most pharmacies carry doughnut-shaped chair cushions that will make sitting more comfortable while you are healing. You'll probably take oral antibiotics for the first ten days to two weeks.

After a week or so, you can become more active. Postpone returning to work, driving, golfing and other sports, and long shopping trips until at least two weeks after the procedure.

You'll return to your doctor to have the Foley catheter removed at

Cyrosurgery for Prostate Cancer

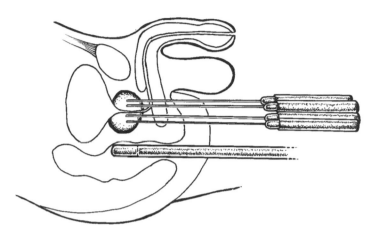

During cryosurgery, an ultrasound probe, inserted in the rectum, produces an image of the prostate gland on a television monitor. The doctor uses this image to guide the cryoprobes into the gland, where the probes freeze tissue.

approximately two weeks. You'll probably have a PSA blood test at three months and every three months after that for two years. Depending on what your PSA does, you may have a biopsy anytime within the first year.

Prostate Cryoablation Advantages

Scholars continually debate the advantages and disadvantages of the various prostate cancer therapies. Cryoablation, being comparatively new, gets its share of criticism as well as praise.

Supporters point out that the cryoablation procedure is not nearly as traumatic for the body as a radical prostatectomy. There is no major incision so it is less invasive, and the frozen tumor does not have to be removed from the body after it is destroyed. Over time, the body's natural defense mechanism simply converts the dead cells to scar tissue. Tumors that are adhered to vital structures, such as major blood vessels, can be destroyed without injuring these structures.

Another advantage of cryosurgery is that all types of cancer cells respond equally to cryoablation, including aggressive prostate tumors—those with high Gleason scores—that are *radioresistant*, not easily destroyed by radiation therapy. In addition, since prostate cryoablation doesn't disrupt the surrounding normal tissue, it can be repeated without additional complications.

Cryosurgery was very satisfactory for me. As far as complications go, I never had any incontinence. I wore a catheter for three or four weeks, which was not uncomfortable; it was easy to tolerate. The procedure really doesn't take a lot out of you.
—Dick, 64

Also, there is some evidence—though further study is needed—that prostate cancer cryoablation patients have a better immune response to their cancers than they did before treatment. Freezing seems to cause the immune system to produce new tumor antibodies, substances the body produces to defend against disease, to fight the cancer. If continued research bears this out, cryosurgery may act as a tumor "vaccine" to strengthen a patient's immune system.

In addition, cryoablation may produce fewer undesirable side effects than other treatments. In a recent study, the researchers used ten years' worth of articles on prostate cancer treatment to compare the various methods. Cryoablation had the lowest range of incontinence rates and the lowest occurrence of rectal complications.

Prostate Cryoablation Disadvantages

The main disadvantage of cryoablation is that only five- and seven-year follow-up data is available. There hasn't been time to compare long-term results of cryoablation with other treatments. Still, nothing in the present data shows the results of cryoablation deteriorating over time.

Finding an Experienced Surgeon

Since cryoablation is a newer form of treatment for prostate cancer, it is important to be aware of certain facts before deciding to undergo this type of treatment. Although 300 surgeons in the United States are currently performing cryoablation, many are still relatively inexperienced. It is therefore extremely important that you find out how many procedures your surgeon has performed. A cryosurgeon should have performed at least 25 procedures; this number is usually considered the minimum needed to be competent. You should also understand that the techniques of cryosurgery can vary from surgeon to surgeon.

Are You a Candidate for Cryoablation?

You may want to talk with your doctor about cryoablation as a primary treatment if your cancer is confined to the prostate, seminal vesicles, and neurovascular bundles, especially if there is a medium to high risk of your cancer recurring, or if you want the lowest possible risk of side effects. You may also be a candidate for prostate cancer cryoablation as salvage therapy after radiation.

Cryotherapy is most effective if your prostate gland weighs 40 grams or less, as measured by ultrasound. If the gland is larger than 40 grams, your doctor may recommend several months of hormone therapy to shrink the gland before attempting cryoablation. (As explained in Chapter 1, the prostate weighs about 20 grams at age 20 and enlarges progressively as you get older.)

Do You Have a Medium to High Risk of Recurrence?

Cryoablation may offer new hope to prostate cancer patients whose cancer is likely to recur even after radical prostatectomy or radiation. There's no sure-fire way to tell whose cancer will come back, but some fairly reliable indicators are stage, grade (Gleason score), and PSA. When those indicators suggest a medium to high risk of prostate cancer recurrence, cryoablation might be effective as a primary therapy.

According to research conducted at two different institutions, medium- and high-risk patients had an 85 percent chance of being disease free at five years when treated with cryoablation as primary therapy. By comparison, rates for similar patients who had radical surgery or radiation were 30 to 60 percent. The reasons may relate to cryoablation's ability to freeze cancers that have escaped from the prostate, the strengthened immunity that cryoablation may give patients, and the ability to repeat cryosurgery if cancer does recur. In these studies, about 15 percent of the patients were retreated.

Cryosurgery as Salvage Therapy after Radiation

Patients whose prostate cancer returns after radiation, but is still confined to prostate, may still be considered curable. Early attempts to use cryoablation as a salvage therapy after radiation were not successful. However, recent advances in cryosurgical technique have met with much greater success. The research data examined men whose cancer was still confined to the prostate. Seventy-five percent of these patients reverted to disease-free status when cryoablation was used as a salvage therapy after radiation failed. However, the complication rate was higher than in patients who had not had previous radiation.

The American Urological Association now supports the use of cryoablation as salvage therapy after radiation, and the Centers for Medicare and Medicaid Services has designated cryoablation as the only treatment specifically approved as a salvage therapy after radiation treatment fails.

The "Male Lumpectomy"

For those men who are more worried about treatment side effects and complications than they are about the cancer itself, cryosurgical lumpectomy—freezing *only* the tumor rather than the entire gland—may be an option, though it is very new and not widely performed in the United States.

The breast-sparing surgery known as *lumpectomy,* which revolu-tionized breast cancer treatment, showed that cancer treatment could be effective while preserving the patient's appearance and, to a great extent, her quality of life. Prostate cancer in men raises many of the same issues that breast cancer does in women. Treatment complications, including impotence and incontinence, can affect a man's self-image every bit as much as the loss of a breast can affect a woman's.

Many men choose watchful waiting over surgery or radiation for prostate cancer because they consider the risks of treatment to be unacceptable. For these men, *cryolumpectomy* to destroy the cancer without sacrificing the entire prostate might be an acceptable middle ground.

This approach isn't for every man with prostate cancer. It wouldn't be effective for men with *multifocal prostate cancer*, in which malig-nancy occurs at several sites within the prostate. But at least one-third of prostate cancer patients, according to some estimates, have *unifocal* disease—a single nodular tumor—and might be candidates for a focal treatment directed at the tumor, rather than the entire gland.

> *It has been six years since my cryosurgery. My PSA is currently 0.25. I feel I have been cured. I now attend numerous prostate support groups and encourage others to consider cryoablation in their search for what is best for them.*
>
> *—George, 74*

Though the procedure is too new for long-term studies, male lumpectomy results to date demonstrate that the approach can control cancer and limit complica-tions. One of the reasons this approach is possible without endangering patients is the unique safety net that cryosurgery offers. If, through regular PSA testing or rebiopsy, remaining cancer is found, doctors can perform cryoablation again to the diseased area.

Risks, Complications, and Side Effects

There is risk of injury to the rectum during cryoablation. The prostate and rectum are separated by a very thin sheet of tissue called

Denonvillier's fascia. A majority of prostate tumors occur in the part of the prostate closest to the rectum, which is why these tumors can sometimes be felt during a rectal exam. If the rectum is accidentally frozen during cryoablation, the result can be a *urethrorectal fistula,* a hole between the digestive and urinary tracts. Should this occur, bacteria escaping from the rectum into the bladder can cause a serious infection and major surgery must be performed to repair the hole. This potential complication underscores the importance of injecting saline into Denonvillier's fascia to separate these two organs.

A predictable side effect of cryoablation is impotence since the neurovascular bundles are usually frozen along with the prostate. All men who undergo cryosurgery for prostate cancer experience impotence immediately after the surgery; about 45 percent regain sexual function. Nerve-sparing cryoablation of the prostate is still in its infancy, but for those who undergo this form of cryoablation, the impotence rate is about 15 percent. Approximately 85 percent regain sexual function.

As stressed in an earlier chapter, men who do experience impotence can still have a sex life. They still have normal sensation and the ability to become sexually aroused and have an orgasm. They're also candidates for drugs such as Viagra, penile implants and injections, which have helped so many men regain the ability to have erections.

It will take a few weeks for you to be able to urinate normally. At first you might have to urinate more often than usual, and you'll probably feel some burning with urination. You may see small flecks of tissue, which were destroyed during cryoablation, in your urine. Very rare after cryoablation of the prostate is severe permanent incontinence, which affects only about 1 percent of patients. The risk of this complication rises, however, if you have had previous radiation or prostate surgery such as TURP.

Expect the tip of the penis to feel numb for a time and the scrotum to be sore and swollen. These are normal, temporary side effects that will probably disappear within a few days.

6

Hormone Therapy

Hormone therapy for prostate cancer works by depriving prostate cells, both cancerous and noncancerous, of the fuel they need to survive and grow. That fuel is testosterone, most of which is manufactured in the testicles.

Until just a few years ago, most doctors delayed starting hormone treatments until symptoms of advanced prostate cancer had become acute, as with bone metastases, for example. The thinking was that, since hormone treatments couldn't cure the cancer and created undesirable side effects, these treatments were best reserved for *palliative* use—improving quality of life and sometimes giving patients another year or two of survival.

Newer studies have shown that starting hormone therapy sooner adds more years with good quality of life, and that hormone treatments are highly useful as therapies along with radical prostatectomy, radiation, and cryoablation. Hormone therapy is still an important palliative treatment.

Scientists are rapidly improving hormone therapy for prostate cancer. Some forms of treatment that had fallen out of favor are getting another look as researchers find ways to counteract their side effects. In this chapter you'll read about a few such therapies, not widely used at present, that nevertheless are still or may soon be part of the prostate cancer treatment arsenal.

How Hormone Therapy Works

Because prostate cells, both normal and cancerous, are fueled by *androgens,* specifically testosterone, scientists have long understood the potential of *androgen deprivation* as a way of controlling prostate cancer. Even when cancer has escaped from the prostate itself, the metastases—whether in the lymph nodes, the bones, or elsewhere in the body—are still essentially prostate cancer cells that can't reproduce without testosterone to feed them.

All hormone therapies work in different ways toward the same goal—to keep testosterone from fueling prostate cancer growth. Hormone therapy drugs can break the testosterone production sequence at any level—keeping testosterone from being made in the first place or blocking its entrance into cancer cells at the end of the cycle.

> *I started hormone therapy three months ago. I've had hot flashes, but they were manageable. I intend to fight on. Life is good, and I believe we can and will win our battles.*
> *— Roy, 58*

When androgen-dependent cells lose access to testosterone, they stop growing and dividing. As they die off, androgen deprivation keeps them from being replaced. In this case, hormone therapy not only stabilizes cancer growth, it also shrinks prostate tumors and the gland itself. If the tumors have been exerting painful pressure on bones or other body structures, that pain is relieved as soon as the tumors start to shrink.

Why then, is androgen deprivation not a cure-all for prostate cancer? Unfortunately, as they grow and reproduce, some prostate cancer cells mutate, becoming *androgen independent*. In effect, they "learn" to survive and thrive without testosterone. Why some men develop a small proportion of androgen-independent cells, whereas other men develop many more, is not well understood. But for those with fewer androgen-independent cells, hormone therapy can work well for many years, even after other treatments have failed. In general, the lower the percentage of androgen-independent cells, the more likely hormone therapy will assist in long-term survival.

Orchiectomy

Among types of hormone therapy, *orchiectomy* or *surgical castration* is one of the fastest acting and least expensive. In a fairly simple procedure, the surgeon makes a small incision in the scrotum, eases the testicles out of their capsules, clamps and seals off the blood vessels with sutures, removes the testicles, and closes the incision. You might not even need general anesthesia. Light sedation and local anesthesia might be all that's required, and you can probably go home the same day or the next.

With the testicles out of commission, in three to twelve hours a man's testosterone drops to *castration level,* the standard against which all other forms of hormone therapy are measured. The adrenal glands, normally responsible for about 5 percent of the androgens circulating through your bloodstream, continue to produce small amounts of testosterone. The significance of those amounts is still being debated. But almost immediately, symptoms such as bone pain begin to subside.

Does Orchiectomy Carry Risks?

The operation itself carries little risk. If it's done right—under sterile conditions and with the blood vessels properly sealed off—neither infection nor bleeding should be a problem. Keep the incision area clean using a hydrogen peroxide–water solution followed by an antibiotic ointment such as Bacitracin. Be alert to signs of infection such as unusual tenderness or redness or pus seeping from the incision. In the extremely unlikely event of excessive bleeding, the scrotum will become enlarged, dark purple, and painful. If this happens, call your doctor, get to a hospital, or call 911, whichever gives you the quickest access to emergency medical treatment.

Recovery from orchiectomy is generally rapid. You'll be advised to avoid heavy lifting, straining, and immersion (no swimming, tub baths, or hot tubs) for one or two weeks.

Advantages and Disadvantages of Orchiectomy

On the plus side, orchiectomy is clearly effective, greatly reducing pain and adding years to the lives of 80 to 90 percent of patients. It is inexpensive, whereas hormone injections to achieve the same results can cost hundreds of dollars a month. On the minus side, your body will change in ways you might expect, since the changes mirror those of menopause in women. In addition to impotence, you could experience hot flashes, breast tenderness or enlargement, loss of muscle tone, reduction in sex drive, and even osteoporosis. Fortunately, doctors have safe and effective ways to counteract most of these side effects. There are even strategies, including implants, for dealing cosmetically with an empty scrotal sac.

Common Chemical Castration Drugs

LHRH Agonists
- leuprolide (Lupron)
- goserelin (Zoladex)
- buserelin (Suprefact)

LHRH Antagonists
- abarelix (Plenaxis)

Nonsteroidal Antiandrogens
- flutamide (Eulexin)
- bicalutamide (Casodex)
- nilutamide (Nilandron)

Chemical Castration

Understandably, many men consider orchiectomy somewhat drastic and opt for *chemical castration*, also called *medical castration*, which can reduce testosterone to castration level within hours or days after treatment starts. Like orchiectomy, chemical castration disconnects the testosterone pipeline, but it uses drugs rather than surgery to do so.

LHRH Agonists

Drugs known as *agonists* stimulate the action of a cell, drug, or hormone. Used in the treatment of prostate cancer, a *luteinizing hormone-releasing hormone (LHRH)* agonist works at the brain level, basically fooling the pituitary gland into stopping production of the hormones that stimulate the testicles to make testosterone. These are the *luteinizing hormone (LH)* and *follicle-stimulating hormone (FSH)*. Usually delivered by injection every three to four months, these drugs are currently the most common therapy for metastatic prostate cancer. Castration level is usually achieved within three to four weeks.

For the first few days after the injection, there's actually a surge, called a *flare*, in testosterone production. Flares temporarily enlarge the prostate and any androgen-dependent tumors and can aggravate prostate cancer symptoms. Flares are short lived, however, and are usually harmless for men whose symptoms are not advanced. However, for men whose symptoms are already distressing and potentially dangerous—bone pain, spinal cord compression, or bladder obstruction, for example—LHRH agonists may be too risky. Orchiectomy or other forms of hormone therapy would probably work better for these men.

Still, studies have shown these drugs to be as effective as orchiectomy in patients with metastatic prostate cancer and who have little problem with flare. Other types of hormone therapy can be combined with LHRH agonists to minimize flare.

LHRH Antagonists

Just as an agonist stimulates a cellular action, a drug known as an *antagonist* blocks an action. Newer drugs, *LHRH antagonists*, block male hormone production and are intended to prevent prostate cancer from growing. They appear to lower testosterone levels more quickly than LHRH agonists and do not cause tumor flare. Studies are in progress to find out whether these drugs work as well as LHRH agonists in managing prostate cancer.

Antiandrogens

This class of drugs works by saturating androgen receptors in the prostate, blocking the access of *dihydrotestosterone (DHT)* and testosterone to those receptors.

Nonsteroidal antiandrogens don't do as good a job of achieving castration level as other drugs, but given for a week or so before LHRH agonists they can reduce or eliminate flare. So antiandrogens are most often given in combination with LHRH agonists rather than alone. One of the side effects in men is breast enlargement and tenderness known as *gynecomastia*. It is preventable with low-dose radiation to the chest before hormone treatments begin. If you're being treated with an antiandrogen and you develop diarrhea, your doctor will likely reduce the dose.

Estrogens

Estrogen, a sex hormone that regulates women's reproduction, has fallen out of favor as a prostate cancer treatment. Its advantages, however, keep researchers in the chase, looking for ways to harness the drug's benefits without all the drawbacks.

In men, estrogen mimics testosterone in the feedback loop. In other words, when estrogen masquerades as testosterone in the bloodstream, it "fools" your brain. The pituitary "thinks" that your testosterone levels are adequate and cuts back production of the testosterone-stimulating hormones LH and FSH. Testosterone then drops to castration level.

Hormone therapy with the synthetic estrogen *diethylstilbestrol (DES)*, as well as other forms of estrogen, once showed great promise in prostate cancer treatment, though today they are seldom used. DES is inexpensive and convenient in tablet form. Unfortunately, at doses high enough to be effective against cancer, estrogens carry unacceptable cardiovascular risks, including heart disease, strokes, and blood clots.

Scientists are seeking ways to combine estrogen with other substances that could neutralize those side effects.

An herbal formula, PC SPES, is something of an anomaly in cancer treatment. It drew the attention and for a time the support of mainstream medical doctors. A mixture of Chinese herbs, PC SPES contains *phytoestrogens*, naturally occurring estrogen-like compounds found in plants.

Though PC SPES may be effective against both androgen-dependent and androgen-independent prostate cancer, independent testing of the product has found traces of prescription drugs. Because of this and other uncertainties surrounding PC SPES, it is no longer available in the United States.

Estrogen treatment is sometimes grouped with other endocrine therapies, all of which have at least some effectiveness against both androgen-independent and androgen-dependent prostate cancers. Among them are P450 enzyme inhibitors (Ketoconazole, HDK), which disrupt hormone production. These therapies are controversial because of potentially dangerous side effects, such as liver damage.

> *At age 74 my PSA went to 10-plus within a six-month period. Biopsies verified I had cancer outside the prostate. I started on hormone drugs to stop the cancer growth and reduce prostate size, allowing me several months to find another solution.*
>
> *—Richard, 70*

Cyproterone Acetate (CPA, Androcur)

Cyproterone acetate (CPA, sold as Androcur) is a steroidal antiandrogen that not only blocks androgen receptors in the prostate but also lowers LH. Because it can cause cardiovascular complications, CPA is not available in the United States, though it is widely used in Canada with LHRH agonists, to prevent flare.

Drug Combinations

Encouraging results have been seen with hormone-therapy combinations, such as the combined androgen blockade in which nonsteroidal antiandrogens are used with orchiectomy or LHRH agonists. This makes sense since it takes both drugs to stop the production of testosterone by both the adrenal glands and the testicles. In general the results of this *combined hormonal therapy* has been impressive enough that this should be the treatment of first choice unless your physician has objections to it.

In some cases, these drugs are used intermittently. *Intermittent hormone therapy* is just what it sounds like—on-again, off-again treatments that are stopped and started based on decreases and increases in PSA levels or troublesome symptoms. Some patients have done well enough after a year of hormone therapy to stop treatments for up to four years before resuming. During this treatment break, men generally become free of the side effects—bone loss, impotence, gynecomastia, hot flashes, and others—that can accompany hormone therapy.

Are You a Candidate for Hormone Therapy?

According to recent evidence, you might well benefit from hormone therapy under any of the following conditions:

- You want to buy time to consider your treatment options.
- You want to decrease the tumor volume before radiation therapy or cryoablation.
- You absolutely refuse to consider invasive treatments such as surgery, brachytherapy, or cryotherapy.
- Your PSA rises significantly after surgery or radiation.

Hormone therapy can also be a primary treatment in older men who may not be strong enough for invasive treatment or who have widespread metastatic disease.

Risks, Complications, and Side Effects of Hormone Therapy

Since not all hormone treatments work the same way, side effects may differ. You might experience impotence, lower sex drive, fatigue, increased cholesterol, hot flashes, anemia, gynecomastia, osteoporosis, emotional changes, and difficulty concentrating. Your voice will not get higher, contrary to popular myth, nor will hormone therapy regrow the hair on your head. Most of these problems disappear or lessen after you stop hormone therapy.

Osteoporosis can take inches off your height and make your bones so brittle they break easily. A new class of drugs called *bisphosphonates* (including Fosamax, Actonel, Aredia, and Zometa) are particularly effective in fighting osteoporosis and may prevent bone metastases. Gynecomastia, as mentioned earlier, can be prevented with low-dose radiation, although this treatment has little effectiveness *after* starting hormone treatment. Low doses of estrogen, pills or patches, work well against hot flashes without causing cardiovascular problems.

Most of the side effects listed here are more uncomfortable or inconvenient than they are dangerous, and most can be alleviated with medication or alternative types of treatment. On the other hand, if you have cardiovascular problems to begin with, if you have liver damage, or if you have metastases that could be dangerously aggravated by the flare phenomenon of LHRH agonists, you will want to approach hormone therapy with caution and frequent monitoring.

Ask your doctor whether hormone treatment would help you as an adjuvant or a neoadjuvant therapy. If you're considering radiation treatment, for example, pretreatment with hormones for up to eight months might make the primary therapy, radiation, more effective by shrinking the prostate and the cancer itself.

7

Chemotherapy

You've probably heard a great deal about chemotherapy as a treatment for cancer. However, until recently it played little part in fighting prostate cancer. Fortunately, research has found new and better uses for chemotherapy in the treatment of prostate cancer, with gentler side effects and with greater potential for helping patients live longer and more comfortably. Improved chemotherapy drugs and techniques offer a variety of new ways to attack cancer cells, and PSA testing allows doctors to test chemotherapy's effectiveness against prostate cancer more accurately than before.

How Chemotherapy Works

Chemotherapy agents, which are often used in conjunction with surgery, radiation, or hormone therapy, are potent chemicals designed to kill cancer cells throughout the body. Chemotherapy drugs work in different ways, depending on the type used. Some prevent *angiogenesis*, the growth of new blood vessels through which cancer can spread. Others arrest cancer cells in different phases of their growth cycles. There are chemotherapy drugs that restore *apoptosis*—the normal cell death process, which cancer cells resist—and those that attack DNA within the genes or keep DNA cells from growing and reproducing.

Doctors once shunned chemotherapy for prostate cancer for a couple of reasons. First, most chemotherapy drugs work much better on fast-growing cancers than on slower growing prostate cancer cells. Second, as chemotherapy agents travel through your body destroying healthy cells as well as cancer cells, they produce unpleasant and sometimes dangerous side effects. For prostate cancer, the questionable benefits didn't seem to be worth the side effects.

These days, however, dozens of chemotherapy drugs are in use and dozens more being tested. There are also new ways of measuring how well these drugs work, along with new medications to address the undesirable side effects of chemotherapy.

Here's more good news about chemotherapy side effects: If you have frequent low doses of cancer-fighting chemicals, you'll likely be more comfortable during chemotherapy—and the treatment might be more effective—than if you have fewer, larger doses. Slow-growing prostate cancer cells require longer exposure time to cancer-fighting chemicals than fast-growing cells. Doctors have found that they can increase exposure time and reduce side effects by administering chemotherapy in, say, daily oral doses or frequent injections.

I am on chemotherapy—three weeks of treatment, one week of rest, three weeks of treatment. My PSA took a nose dive and is still dropping. My doctor says there is a good chance of remission. I'm spending all my spare time with my grandchildren.

— Tim, 68

One way of giving you frequent low doses at an effective level is through a painless *venous access device,* such as a Port-a-Cath—a small computerized pump implanted under the skin, usually on the chest. A small plastic disk, called a *port,* on the skin's surface connects to a tube threaded into a vein, supplying low doses of chemotherapy agents to minimize side effects and increase exposure time.

As a bonus, these devices greatly reduce the risk of *extravasation injury,* damage that occurs around the injection site when chemotherapy drugs leak into nearby tissues. If extravasation injury does occur, your doctor can prescribe a medicinal cream to rub onto the injured area.

Preparing for Chemotherapy

Your chemotherapy drugs may be given as a pill or in liquid form by injection, or by an IV drip, an *infusion*, through a catheter or port. If you are having oral (by mouth) chemotherapy, you can probably do your own treatments at home. Chemotherapy injections and infusions, however, are usually done in a clinic or hospital. Your treatments can take from a few minutes to several hours, depending on the drug, the dose, and the method used. Some doctors admit chemotherapy patients for overnight observation in a hospital after their first treatment.

I had chemotherapy through a port-a-cath for 17 weeks. I was all set to deal with hair loss, but there wasn't any! I had very little nausea and could still go to work. That was eight years ago, and I'm still ticking.
—Pat, 60

Before beginning chemotherapy, your doctor might order blood tests, X-rays and other imaging studies, and biopsies. These tests can help the doctor locate metastases and determine whether your blood is healthy enough for chemotherapy at that time. The better your overall health when chemotherapy begins, the fewer troublesome side effects you're likely to have.

If you need dental work, your doctor might suggest getting it done at least two weeks before your treatments start. Having dental work during the course of chemotherapy is difficult for at least two reasons: You're more prone to infection then, and chemotherapy can cause mouth sores. Why mouth sores? As mentioned earlier, chemotherapy kills fast-growing cells, and the cells in the lining of the mouth grow rapidly.

Before your chemotherapy begins, your doctor might start you on antinausea drugs and recommend that you drink a lot of fluids and avoid spicy and fatty foods. You will probably be advised not to eat or drink at all during the two hours before your chemotherapy treatment.

Chemotherapy Side Effects

Unlike radiation, which targets specific areas where cancer has been found, chemotherapy's action is systemic, meaning that it affects your entire body. As noted earlier, systemic chemotherapy drugs can attack both normal and malignant cells anywhere in your body. The drugs target primarily fast-growing or rapidly dividing cells, such as those in bone marrow, hair follicles, and the reproductive and digestive systems. That's why your hair might fall out and you might feel nauseated at times.

Your doctor will talk with you about the side effects of the particular drug or combination of drugs being used, and about medications and other ways to lessen or eliminate these side effects. Today there are treatments to counteract nearly every negative side effect.

If the list of chemotherapy side effects seems long and overwhelming, please keep a few things in mind. First, most of these conditions will return to normal when your body has had a chance to recover after chemotherapy. Second, there are now many chemotherapy drugs to choose from, so if one is particularly troublesome, your doctor can likely switch to a different one. Third, there are many ways to alleviate these side effects, including prescription drugs, over-the-counter products, and lifestyle adjustments. Your doctor and your support group can be tremendously helpful, so never feel you must suffer in silence. The sooner you describe what's troubling you, the sooner an effective remedy can be supplied.

Digestive Tract Side Effects

Chemotherapy can cause a variety of side effects, almost always temporary, throughout the digestive

---

Chemotherapy Agents for Prostate Cancer

- mitoxantrone (Novantrone)
- estramustine phosphate (Emcyt)
- etoposide (Vepsid)
- paclitaxel (Taxol)
- docetaxel (Taxotere)
- doxorubicin (Adriamycin)
- vinblastine (Velban)

tract. Nausea, vomiting, constipation, diarrhea, loss of appetite, and mouth and throat sores can afflict patients undergoing chemotherapy. Not everyone experiences all these side effects, which can vary with the type of drug, the dose, and the frequency and duration of chemotherapy.

Scientists continue to formulate new chemotherapy drugs, some of them nausea free, and new ways of giving these drugs that decrease the side effects. And there's a great deal you and your doctor can do to prevent, minimize, or eliminate side effects.

Eating a balanced diet, high in fiber and low in fat, is one of the most important steps you can take to counter digestive side effects. Drink plenty of fluids, especially water. You might want to avoid acidic liquids, such as coffee, some teas, citrus fruit juices, and tomato juice, since these substances can be hard on your stomach even without the aggravating effect of chemotherapy. Alcoholic beverages can also worsen digestive tract side effects.

Many adults are lactose intolerant; their bodies lack the enzyme lactase, needed to digest milk sugar (lactose). For these people, milk and milk products can cause diarrhea or constipation, especially during chemotherapy. You should be able to tolerate yogurt, however, which contains beneficial bacteria that basically predigest the lactose for you.

Sometimes all it takes is an over-the-counter product such as Imodium-AD for diarrhea or milk of magnesia for constipation. If these don't work, prescription drugs can help.

Diarrhea, anorexia, and vomiting can be dangerous, causing you to become malnourished or dehydrated. It's important to tell your doctor if you're experiencing any of these symptoms. Don't assume they're just part of the treatment process.

Damage to Blood and Bone Marrow

The large bones in your body have soft, spongy centers called *bone marrow* where your blood cells are made. These cells reproduce rapidly in the bone marrow, so they are especially vulnerable to chemo-therapy drugs. It's extremely important to protect these cells, because they do some of the most important work in your body.

While you're on chemotherapy, your doctor will order blood tests to monitor the most serious potential side effects from damage to bone marrow and blood cell production.

White blood cells (WBCs) fight infection. If you have an infection—anything from an abscessed tooth to pneumonia—your WBC count goes up. Chemotherapy destroys white blood cells before they can reproduce, causing a low WBC count. Symptoms can include chills or fever, nasal congestion, coughing, shortness of breath, and swelling and tenderness at the site of an injury.

Red blood cells carry oxygen to every cell in your body. The oxygen enables these cells to produce energy. If you are anemic, you will likely be unusually tired and irritable. You may experience headaches, dizziness, shortness of breath, and even chest pain.

Platelets are responsible for blood clotting. If you have a low platelet count, you may have nosebleeds, you might bruise easily, and small cuts might bleed excessively. If your platelet count is extremely low, you could even have internal bleeding. Blood-thinning products, such as those containing aspirin or ibuprofen, decrease platelet production. Ask your doctor which medications you should avoid.

My husband has had five weeks of radiation, hormone shots every three months, implanted radioactive seeds, and is just starting chemotherapy. We have been married 42 years, and I am happy to have him the way he is now. We are both in our early 60s and love just holding each other.
—Senyour, wife

In the recent past, these blood-related side effects sent patients to the hospital for round-the-clock monitoring. It was often necessary to delay chemotherapy or needed surgery. These drastic measures, along with blood transfusions, are less common today thanks to new synthetic versions of naturally occurring growth factors, which stimulate blood cell formation. Several commonly used ones include:

- The drug epoetin (Procrit) can stimulate your bone marrow to manufacture red blood cells, making transfusions unnecessary.

- Another newer drug, opralvekin (Neumega), stimulates platelet production in bone marrow.

- Neupogen and Leukine are colony stimulating factors, drugs that stimulate white cell production, greatly reducing infections.

Hair Loss and Nail Changes

As chemotherapy destroys cancer cells, it also destroys the rapidly reproducing cells responsible for hair and nail growth. Once chemotherapy is completed, these cells usually recover and your hair and nails go back to normal. Often, the new hair growth is a slightly different color or texture than it was before chemotherapy, but the change is usually temporary.

It usually takes a few weeks after you begin chemotherapy for your hair to start thinning. Some patients decide to shave off all their hair at this point, in part because wigs stay on better and are more comfortable on a bald scalp.

Your insurance may cover the cost of a wig or hair prosthesis. The latter is basically a wig that is custom designed and fitted so it looks more natural. You may simply choose to go bald and enjoy the temporary freedom from washing and cutting your hair. Do wear a cap when you're outdoors to prevent sunburn.

At this time, little can be done to prevent chemotherapy-induced hair loss—not a dangerous side effect but sometimes a distressing one. There are no drugs, food supplements, or hair treatment products that can prevent it, despite the claims that appear on the Internet and in magazine ads. Your doctor and your support group can suggest ways to cope with hair loss.

Some chemotherapy patients never experience problems with their hair or nails. Most, however, find that their hair gets very thin or brittle, eventually breaking off near the roots or falling out altogether. Your fingernails and toenails won't fall off, but white bands might appear on them and they may also change color. Keeping them short and filed smooth not only will improve their appearance, it will keep you from accidentally tearing a nail or scratching yourself.

Skin Changes

During chemotherapy, your skin may be itchy and dry, you might notice a rash, you could be more susceptible to sunburn, and you might develop sores or blisters—all normal to a degree. Be sure to let your doctor know if these conditions are severe, however, because skin abnormalities can signal an allergic reaction to the chemotherapy drugs. To prevent infection, immediately call your doctor's attention to any open sores.

Some chemo patients just don't feel up to their normal routine, especially if they work full time. I help them negotiate things at work, like telecommuting if possible, or flexible scheduling, or invoking the Family Medical Leave Act.

— Donna, social worker

If your skin is flaking, your bedding harbors dead skin and bacteria, so change your sheets often. Take warm but not hot showers and baths. Baking soda in your bath water can minimize itching. Ask your doctor about taking vitamin E or zinc supplements. Your doctor might also recommend skin products containing aloe vera or oatmeal (such as Alpha Keri). Use mild skin cleansers, shampoos, and laundry products (such as Dreft and Ivory Snow, which are gentle enough for babies' sensitive skin). Wear sunscreen, at least 15 SPF, any time you go outdoors. Drink plenty of fluids to hydrate your skin, and avoid extremes of heat or cold.

Mouth and Throat Sores

Mouth and throat sores can be aggravated both by a low WBC count and by chemotherapy's effects on your digestive system. It's a good idea to brush your teeth often with a soft toothbrush and avoid mouthwash that contains alcohol, which can be too harsh for the sensitive tissues in your mouth. Some doctors recommend rinsing your mouth with a mild salt-water solution, while others claim that salt can worsen mouth sores. Avoid hard, crunchy foods and those with high acid content (tomatoes, citrus fruits), a lot of salt or spices, and caffeine. Don't smoke or chew tobacco.

Nervous System Changes

Some chemotherapy drugs can damage the nervous system and may have an effect on the way your brain functions. Immediately report symptoms to your doctor such as headache, confusion, depression, fever, numbness or tingling in the extremities, dry mouth, vision problems, and ringing in the ears. Prescription drugs such as amifostine (Ethyol) may prevent many of these problems. Doctors sometimes prescribe antidepressants such as amitriptyline (Elavil), desipramine (Norpramin), or nortriptyline (Pamelor) for chemotherapy-related depression and other symptoms. Anticonvulsants, including carbamazepine (Tegretol) and gabapentin (Neurotin), can alleviate pain that stems from nervous system damage. Increasingly, doctors are recommending acupuncture and acupressure, which may effectively relieve pain for many patients not helped by drugs.

Neuropathy, tingling and loss of sensation in the hands or feet, is a common side effect during prolonged use of some chemotherapy drugs. Medications are being developed to counteract this effect. Ask your doctor about using folic acid, one of the B vitamins, shown by numerous studies to be effective against chemotherapy-induced neuropathy.

Kidney and Liver Damage

A few chemotherapy drugs can cause liver or kidney damage. You'll have blood work periodically to check your kidney and liver function. If kidney or liver damage is suspected, your doctor may switch you to another chemotherapy drug. Some prescription drugs can prevent such damage. Sodium thiosulfate, for example, may protect both the kidneys and the bone marrow.

8

Life after Treatment for Prostate Cancer

If you're recovering from prostate cancer treatment or you're having hormone therapy, your body has changed, and may continue to change, in ways you might find confusing, embarrassing, even depressing. Take heart. There's help for you—medical, spiritual, and emotional—though for many men, the most difficult thing is to ask for it.

Think of all the *giving* you've done in your life—to family, friends, your job, perhaps your place of worship—and allow yourself to *take* for a change. Take advantage of the many resources that are available to you from organizations, medical professionals, family, friends, books and tapes, pastors and counselors. Take some time for yourself and your loved ones. Take time to do the things you've always wanted to do. Be kind to yourself. Pamper yourself. Many men report that they enjoy life more because they learned so much about living life and enjoying it to the fullest.

Coping Emotionally

Support Groups

Some of the most powerful support available comes from men like you—prostate cancer survivors who are grateful to be alive. These men gather in community centers and hospital meeting rooms, or in online discussion groups, to share their stories, draw strength from each other, and learn about prostate cancer treatment advances. More than anyone else, they know what you've been through and what you're facing. They can recommend physicians and therapists, books and videos, organizations and other resources. With their help you can learn to talk about your illness and the effect it's having on your life.

There's at least one more good reason to get involved with a support group. Studies have consistently shown that cancer patients in strong support groups live longer. *Strong* is a key word here. Most support groups are upbeat and encouraging. A few are dominated by pessimists, naysayers, or people who just won't stop talking. If you find yourself in one of these, seek out another one. The last thing you need is to surround yourself with gloom and doom, especially when there's so much to feel good about.

How to Find a Support Group

First, ask your urologist. Actually, you probably won't even have to ask. Physicians know the value of such support and routinely steer their patients toward relevant support groups. You can also get local meeting information online or by calling or writing the American Cancer Society or the prostate cancer support organizations Man to Man and Us Too! For details on these and other sources of information and support, see the Resources section in the back of this book.

Spiritual Resources

Some men gain a sense of well-being in prayer or fellowship groups, yoga classes, and meditation gatherings. Through the ages, people have relied on prayer, pastoral counseling, and close-knit religious communities to help them through illness and other difficulties. Many members of the clergy in nearly every denomination have received training in pastoral counseling. A growing number of physicians actively recommend these spiritual resources to their patients, not only because of their own faith experiences but also because of new research that validates the role of prayer and church attendance in healing and prolonging life.

Help for Depression

It's not uncommon for men to get depressed, anxious, or both, when their prostate cancer is diagnosed. You might have been devastated when you found out you had prostate cancer, and thrilled when you learned about curative treatment options. Maybe you were nervous before surgery or radiation, but depressed in the aftermath when your energy flagged and your bowels didn't work right. Perhaps you were anxious when you wondered if that ache or that slightly elevated PSA meant your cancer had returned.

In some cases, prostate cancer is like living with diabetes. One never gets rid of it but can live with it and control the disease well.
—*Dr. Arthur Centeno*
Urologist

Talk to your doctor right away. Don't delay getting help for depression or anxiety. A cheerful outlook is your best friend. With medication, counseling, or a combination of the two, you can find the tools that are so important right now to take care of yourself, stay informed, and participate fully and joyfully in life.

Talk to Your Partner

If you have a mate, hopefully you have emotional support and can share your fears and joys. Perhaps you have a close friend or relative you can count on to be there for you. Maybe you're a person who has held things in all your life. Perhaps you've thought that being "strong" meant dealing with your problems on your own. Maybe it's time to let down your defenses and stop being a hero.

Please realize that your prostate cancer affects those who love you almost as much as it affects you, even if you don't talk about it openly. Couples who go through big changes together, keeping the lines of communication open, usually emerge stronger and closer than they were before. This is an opportunity for your relationship to grow.

Take your spouse or partner with you to doctor's appointments and support group meetings. Share your hopes and fears. You're entitled to them. Discuss treatment options, side effects, the possibility of impotence or incontinence, and the information you gather. Two heads really are better than one when you're trying to solve a problem, make a decision, or overcome anxiety.

Your Children, Other Family Members, Friends, and Co-workers

What should you tell the kids? Many counselors recommend a balance between honesty and reassurance, depending on your children's ages, and advise against trying to protect them by keeping them in the dark. Grown children are likely to be hurt if they're deprived of a chance to help and support their dad, and even very young children know and become anxious when something disquieting is going on.

What you say to other people depends on your relationship with them and their need to know. Don't worry that you're burdening people when you tell them about your illness. Most people are eager to help when they can, even if it's just by listening. On the other hand, your fellow cocktail party guests would probably prefer not to hear the toe-curling details of your orchiectomy or brachytherapy procedure.

When people ask how they can help, tell them. Do you need transportation to the doctor's office or the hospital? Do you just want someone to listen? Let them know! If they genuinely care about you, you'll be doing them a favor by letting them contribute to your well-being.

Your Doctor Can Help

Your doctor and his or her staff can give you information, referrals, and encouragement. Be assured that your urologist and probably your primary care doctor have heard every embarrassing question in the book, from "What kind of undergarment is best for leakage?" to "What kind of penile implant is most 'natural' and safest?" If you're not completely honest with your doctor, you risk losing access to a drug or procedure that could make your life a lot more enjoyable.

Coping with Incontinence

Some degree of incontinence is likely after radical prostatectomy, radiation therapy, or cryotherapy. It's almost always temporary, though in some cases it can be a problem for years. In the case of radiation therapy, incontinence may get worse over time because radiation-damaged cells can't repair themselves as other cells do.

Bladder control in healthy men depends on the *urinary sphincter* muscles at the bladder neck and below the bladder around the urethra. Prostate surgery or radiation can damage or weaken these muscles so that they can no longer keep urine from leaking out of the bladder.

Prostate cancer treatment usually causes *stress urinary incontinence*, involuntary leaking of urine when you cough, sneeze, laugh, or get up out of a chair. After radical prostatectomy, more than 95 percent of patients regain continence, many fairly quickly, though it can take up to three years. Less common with prostate cancer are *urge incontinence*, when you can't get to the bathroom in time, and *overflow incontinence*, when normal urine flow is blocked and the bladder is always full.

Medications for Incontinence

Depending on the type of incontinence you have, your doctor might prescribe simple decongestants, antidepressants, or other drugs to help you regain urinary retention. Drugs are usually the first line of defense in treating incontinence.

Decongestants, which may tighten the urethral muscles, are often prescribed for stress incontinence. These drugs are also called *alpha-adrenergic agonists* and contain ingredients such as ephedrine and pseudoephedrine that are found in nonprescription decongestants and appetite suppressants. If you have high blood pressure, heart disease, diabetes, hyperthyroidism, or glaucoma, you should not take alpha-adrenergic agonists.

For urge incontinence, *anticholinergic agents*—oxybutynin (Ditropan), hyoscyamine (Levbid, Cytospaz), or tolterodine (Detrol)—normally used to treat Parkinson's disease, can help by delaying the urge to urinate and allowing the bladder to hold more urine. Patients have complained about unpleasant side effects—dry eyes and mouth, constipation, and rapid heartbeat—but newer versions of these drugs may be much easier to tolerate.

Tricyclic antidepressants such as imipramine (Tofranil) and amitriptyline (Elavil, Vanatrip, Endep) can help control stress incontinence by tightening the bladder neck muscles. They are not prescribed for people with heart disease and can cause a host of side effects, from dizziness and sweating to dry mouth, headache, constipation, and ringing in the ears. Possible, though uncommon, are more serious side effects, including seizures, heart attack, high blood pressure, and allergic reactions. These drugs can also do their job too well, causing urinary retention.

> *I just saw the doctor for my three-year checkup. Once again , my PSA is less than 0.1. Woohooo! It's always a huge relief when he walks in and says, "Your numbers look good."*
> —Paul, 66

Exercises for Incontinence

One of the best and easiest ways, and certainly the cheapest way, to overcome or diminish the incontinence problem is with *Kegel exercises,* also called *pelvic floor exercises.* These are so simple you can do them almost anywhere. Simply tighten your pelvic muscles, keep them tight for about 10 seconds, and then release.

You use your pelvic muscles many times a day. They're the muscles you use to keep from urinating before you can get to the bathroom. To practice, try stopping the urine stream after you've begun urinating. Some doctors tell their prostate cancer patients to do Kegels for five minutes twenty or so times each day and to start doing them even before treatment. After treatment, keep up this regimen until you're no longer troubled with incontinence.

Your doctor may refer you for physical therapy for help rehabilitating your pelvic muscles. You might not think Kegel exercises would be difficult to master, but it's surprisingly easy to do them wrong. It's important to tighten only the pelvic muscles, not the buttocks or the abdominal or thigh muscles. Some physical therapists use biofeedback to teach the proper way to do Kegel exercises. Biofeedback to reinforce pelvic floor exercises is easy and painless. You'll be hooked up to a machine that lights up or gives another clear signal when you do the exercise correctly. As you try to repeat that response, you get better and better at the exercise until it becomes second nature.

The Male Sling

This new procedure, in which a strip of abdominal or synthetic tissue is surgically placed in the pelvis to compress the urethra, can usually be done on an outpatient basis. Although the sling material is literally screwed to the pubic bone, the procedure can take less than half an hour and requires only a two-inch incision between the scrotum and the rectum. The procedure is not yet widely available, but early studies have shown improvement in 80 percent of the men treated. Many doctors predict that the male sling will become the treatment of choice for male urinary incontinence.

The Condom Catheter

A condom catheter is a simple device that drains leaked urine from the penis. The condom, usually latex, is attached to the penis with adhesive. Also attached to the sheath is a plastic tube that leads to a bag taped to the leg. The urine stays in the attached leg bag until it is emptied.

If you are allergic to latex, the condom catheter probably isn't for you. Many doctors recommend against the device for other reasons as well. Besides being a crutch that can prevent men from working to regain urinary control, the condom catheter can cause urinary tract infections and other problems. If you want to use the condom catheter, do so only under your doctor's supervision and only for brief outings, since the bag must be emptied every thirty minutes.

Penile Clamps

An externally worn penile clamp (Cunningham clamp) can be effective in controlling incontinence. This clamp is simply worn over the penis and places external pressure on the urethra, stopping leakage. When used as prescribed, these clamps can safe and convenient. Clamps are inexpensive and can usually be obtained from your urologist.

I have struggled with incontinence. Now, 16 months after surgery, I seem to be getting better and better. If I'm religious about doing my Kegels twice a day, I do better.

—John, 62

Artificial Urinary Sphincter

If you have lingering incontinence, consider an artificial urinary sphincter, which involves a simple surgical procedure. It can be done on an outpatient basis or with an overnight hospital stay. The procedure is successful up to 90 percent of the time and carries minimal risk. The surgeon will simply place a small balloon in your lower abdomen, an inflatable cuff around the urethra, and a pump in the scrotum.

When the cuff contains fluid it compresses the urethra so that urine can't escape. When you want to urinate, you squeeze the pump a few times. Activating the pump causes the fluid to flow from the cuff to the balloon. After you urinate, the fluid will flow back into the cuff.

As with any minor surgery, there's a slight risk of bleeding or infection. Rare complications can include urinary retention and malfunction or breakage of the device. The artificial sphincter is not a good option for older men, for men who have had radiation therapy, or for those who have vascular disease.

Collagen Injections

Collagen is a natural protein that's commonly used in cosmetic procedures to plump up facial skin and diminish fine lines and wrinkles. It acts similarly when injected into the tissues around the bladder neck to prevent urine leakage out of the bladder. Only men with mild incontinence benefit from collagen injections, which have to be repeated—two or three times at the beginning and again if the leakage comes back. It's a simple outpatient procedure, however, and collagen injections are generally effective for a few years, although effectiveness varies from a few months to many years.

Your doctor will do a skin test to make sure you're not allergic to the collagen, which is derived from cattle. This is a very important precaution, as an allergic reaction could be life threatening. If you've had a radical prostatectomy followed by radiation therapy, collagen injections will not work for you; the injections don't have the "bulking up" effect on the bladder neck.

Incontinence Undergarments

In every drugstore you'll find shelves full of disposable pads and underpants for adults with incontinence. There's a great variety of these products, some made specifically for men. They're very useful, even necessary, immediately after a radical prostatectomy. You probably don't relish the idea of prowling the store aisles looking for the perfect incontinence product, but reassure yourself that it's just a short-term measure and keep doing your Kegels. Ask your doctor which product he or she recommends. Change your pad or undergarment often to avoid odor and chafing.

Coping with Impotence

Every medical treatment for prostate cancer carries a risk of temporary or permanent impotence. It's impossible to know before treatment which men will become impotent and for how long. Even among men in their forties who have the nerve-sparing radical prostatectomy, with both neurovascular bundles preserved, and who had good erections before surgery, 10 percent remain impotent afterward.

Normally, when you start to get an erection, blood flows into the chambers in the penis. It is the blood in these chambers that keeps the penis erect. While you're aroused, the blood vessels are sealed off and the blood can't flow back out. This process may not work well, or at all, after prostate cancer treatment. Impotence occurs when the blood supply or nerve pathways to the penis are damaged. This damage is present to some extent with prostate surgery, radiation, and cryosurgery.

I didn't believe my doctor when he said I could enjoy sex without having an erection. Boy, was I wrong. My wife and I both did our homework, and our sex life is better than ever.
— *Drew, 62*

Hormone therapy causes impotence in an entirely different way, by eliminating testosterone, the hormone that governs male sexuality, from the body. Men who are having hormone therapy for prostate cancer not only become impotent, they lose interest in sex. There is no way to restore potency or sex drive to men who have been surgically castrated with orchiectomy. Men who are undergoing chemical castration, the purpose of hormone therapy, may regain potency when hormone treatments are stopped.

Some men hope to be spared the problem of impotence by delaying treatment as long as possible or foregoing it altogether. These men need to understand that impotence can occur without treatment. In fact, impotence is as much a complication of the disease as it is of the treatment. In addition, 25 percent of men will be impotent by age 65 with or without prostate cancer. Impotence can be a result of diabetes, hypertension, and other disorders, as well as medications, alcohol, smoking, and psychological conditions.

Fortunately, a great deal can be done to help men who have some degree of impotence. Please keep in mind that the word *impotence* refers only to the inability to have an erection. Other parts of the sexual process—libido (sexual desire), ejaculation, and orgasm—are separate. If you are impotent, you can usually continue to enjoy sex and have orgasms.

I was getting up to urinate five or six times a night. The doctor found bladder-neck stricture, which he repaired in an outpatient surgery. Two years after RP surgery, I have no leakage and no problems with urine flow.
—Mac, 60

Better than any device or procedure to restore erections is trust and communication between you and your partner. Be willing to talk openly and to experiment with techniques you both find enjoyable, whether or not they produce an erection.

Drugs for Impotence

The availability of Viagra (sildenafil citrate) and similar drugs has been a boon to prostate cancer patients and other men with impotence or erectile dysfunction. These drugs, called *PDE-5 inhibitors,* work by blocking an enzyme, phosphodiesterase type 5, found in penile tissues. When the enzyme is blocked, the smooth muscles of the penis can relax to allow blood to flow in.

Newer drugs, Levitra (vardenafil) and Cialis (tadalafil), are similar to Viagra and work well for a majority of men. Your doctor will likely tell you to start taking one of these drugs about four to eight weeks after your treatment, just prior to resuming intercourse.

These medications are not aphrodisiacs. They won't help you become aroused. You have to provide the libido; the drug can help supply the erection.

Most men tolerate PDE-5 inhibitors well, but there are some men who should never take them. If you have coronary artery disease, get clearance from your cardiologist before using the drug. If you're taking medicine containing nitrates (such as nitroglycerine or isosorbides), Viagra and similar drugs are not for you. The combination can cause a dangerous drop in blood pressure.

Side effects, though uncommon, can include headache, flushing, indigestion, runny nose, diarrhea, dizziness, and a temporary blue haze or other eyesight disturbance.

Penile Injections

Less unpleasant than they sound, penile injections are actually an easy, painless, and effective way to achieve a normal erection. Using a small syringe with a very fine needle, you'll inject a *vasodilator*, a drug that widens blood vessels, into the penis shaft. The vasodilator opens the blood vessels and relaxes the smooth muscles of the penis. Within ten to twenty minutes, both chambers fill with blood, giving you an erection that lasts thirty minutes to two hours.

I wasn't a candidate for nerve-sparing surgery, but I've been on Viagra since a few months after the operation, and I don't have any trouble with erections.
—Clayton, 60

If you have heart disease, ask your doctor if vasodilators are safe for you. This technique is not for you if for some reason you're unable to give yourself the injection, whether because of squeamishness, poor eyesight, or poor coordination.

It's important that you take the lowest effective dose possible. If the dosage is too high, you could have a prolonged erection that could actually become dangerous. Other side effects can include very small blood clots, burning pain after the injection, damage to the urethra, and

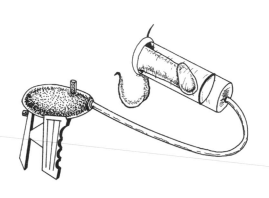

A penile pump is used externally to make blood flow into the shaft and tip of the penis, causing an erection.

fibrous tissue buildup in the corpora cavernosa. Infection, if you've taken sanitary precautions, should never be a problem.

Finally, you may have heard about men who take testosterone injections to help restore sexual function. However, no reputable doctor will prescribe testosterone for you if you are at risk for or being treated for prostate cancer. Testosterone won't produce the desired effect and it could spur the growth of cancerous cells in your body.

Vacuum Erection Devices

A vacuum erection device is basically an airtight tube that you place over your lubricated penis. When you activate the attached pump, it creates a vacuum that draws blood into your penis. To keep the blood from flowing right back out, there's a rubber ring that slides off the tube and onto the base of the penis. These rings come in different sizes. If you have the right size, it won't be uncomfortable.

Vacuum erection devices are safe and effective. You can use them as often as you like, but you must remove the ring after thirty minutes to restore healthy blood flow.

Penile Implants

There are several types of penile implants, or prostheses, all of which work well to produce erections in men who would otherwise be unable to have them. They are inserted into the penis surgically, under anesthetic, through a small incision in the scrotum. Some models have a reservoir, which is implanted in the abdomen, and a pump implanted in the scrotum. The procedure can be done on an outpatient basis or with an overnight stay in the hospital. All implants create a slight increase in penile diameter.

The simplest and least expensive are mechanical, made of flexible materials that keep the penis rigid, but can be bent for urination and to appear natural under clothing. More complex implants are inflatable and, in principle, much like an artificial sphincter. The surgeon implants a fluid reservoir and a cylinder in the penis. When you activate the device, it transfers fluid from the reservoir to the cylinder, creating an erection.

In general, the more sophisticated the device the more likely it is to malfunction, although all models are generally reliable. There are slight risks of infection, scarring, or damage to the two chambers which run the length of the penis.

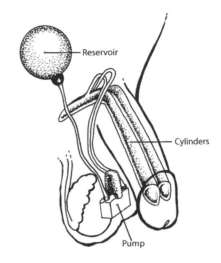

Penile implants are a consideration if other measures fail to produce erections. Long-term data shows penile implants to be highly effective and reliable.

Men often worry that penile implants made of silicone will cause problems similar to those of women who had silicone breast implants a few decades ago. This is simply not the case. There have been a few instances of the body rejecting the device, in which case it is simply removed.

After Prostate Cancer: Follow-Up Care

You'll need to see your doctor regularly to have a PSA blood test and a urinalysis to check for blood in the urine. Your PSA should be 0.0 after surgery, although a PSA of 0.1 or 0.2 shouldn't alarm you, as lab tests have a slight margin of error. After radiation therapy, your PSA will drop slowly, ideally to below 0.5.

Expect to see your doctor three or four times during the first year after treatment, two or three times a year for the next few years, and once or twice a year thereafter, if things are going well. A slight rise in your PSA on one of these visits needn't mean trouble. Your doctor may repeat the test in a couple of months.

After your primary treatment for prostate cancer, your doctor might recommend a diet and exercise regimen to discourage the return of cancer and make you healthier and more energetic at the same time. A high-fiber, low-fat diet can prevent or improve many medical conditions. Ask your doctor to refer you to a nutritionist who can help you streamline a diet according to your preferences and needs.

If Cancer Recurs

Anyone who has had cancer knows what it's like to worry about a recurrence. For a while at least, every little symptom can set alarm bells ringing. You don't want to live every day in a state of heightened anxiety, but you're wise to be concerned and check with your doctor when your body sends you signals you don't understand.

As is true with the initial diagnosis of prostate cancer, the earlier a recurrence is discovered, the better the chance of successfully managing the disease. Your doctor will be alert to any PSA increase. If the PSA continues to rise, it probably means the cancer has returned. A rapid increase signals an aggressive cancer.

This is by no means good news, but there are many avenues of treatment for men whose prostate cancer reappears. A question that doctors still don't agree on is when to start salvage therapy, a treatment after the primary treatment has failed.

Salvage Therapy

Many doctors will recommend salvage radiation treatments if cancer recurs after radical prostatectomy, possibly while your PSA is between 1.0 and 2.0. If your primary treatment was radiation (EBRT or brachytherapy), your doctor may want to start hormone therapy or cryotherapy at the point where your PSA is between 3.0 and 4.0.

Hormone treatments probably won't get rid of your cancer altogether, but they can prolong your life and improve your quality of life for many years.

Performing a salvage prostatectomy after radiation is not unheard of, but it can be dangerous and difficult. Because of tissue damage, there's a good chance of injury to the rectal wall. The patient might require a permanent *colostomy,* a surgical procedure in which the large intestine is routed to an opening in the body through which fecal waste passes into an external bag. He might also be permanently incontinent.

Eventually, prostate cancer can spread through the lymph system and to the bones and elsewhere. Symptoms of metastatic cancer are many and varied—fatigue, weight loss, bone pain, loss of appetite, anemia, and others. With bone loss comes the risk of pathologic fractures, bones that break practically on their own, especially the weight-bearing bones of the hips and thighs.

I talked with my wife about the risk of impotence, and she said, "We've been married 47 years and have had all the sex we need. It's more important to me that you're here and you're healthy."

—Bob, 75

Palliative Care

If the disease cannot be stopped, the purpose of treatment becomes palliative, intended to keep patients as comfortable as possible. Spot radiation, localized EBRT to painful bones, can shrink tumors and relieve pain for several weeks or months. Injections of radioactive materials, strontium-89 (Metastron) or radium-223, target cancer in the bones and provide relief for up to six months. These injections can create a drop in blood production in the bone marrow, necessitating blood transfusions. For 48 hours after an injection, it's important to dispose of urine in the same way other radioactive materials are disposed of.

Spot radiation can also prevent spinal cord compression. This is a very serious condition that, if untreated, can lead to paralysis. Remedies include steroid drugs, surgical decompression, and orchiectomy.

There is no need for any man to be in continuous pain from prostate cancer. Historically, doctors and other health care professionals were afraid to over-prescribe pain medication for fear of causing addiction or serious side effects. Patients have often cooperated with this reluctance by not asking for painkillers no matter how bad they felt.

Today there's new awareness of the unnecessary suffering cancer patients have endured, and patients and their loved ones are being encouraged to make their needs known, loud and clear. There is no such thing as pain that is unresponsive to medication. Painkillers range from mild (nonsteroidal anti-inflammatory drugs, or NSAIDs) to morphine strength, and anyone who is in great pain is entitled to take advantage of the many remedies available.

Other Approaches to Treatment

Nontraditional approaches can be effective, as well, to supplement standard medical care. Biofeedback, meditation, relaxation techniques, hypnosis, acupuncture, and acupressure not only help patients relax and improve their outlook, they've earned the respect of the scientific community, as well.

At any point in your treatment, speak up about things that concern you—pain or even mild discomfort, symptoms that alarm you, changes in the way your body functions. Don't assume that these problems just come with the territory. Scientists have spent years developing solutions for the very problems you may be having.

Appendix

Simplified Summary of TNM Staging System
for Prostate Cancer

T = Tumor   **N** = Nodes   **M** = Metastases

Stage T1

Tumor is microscopic and confined to prostate but is undetectable by a digital rectal exam (DRE) or by ultrasound. Usually discovered by PSA tests or biopsies.

Stage T2

Tumor is confined to prostate and can be detected by DRE or ultrasound.

Stage T3 or T4

In stage T3, the cancer has spread to tissue adjacent to the prostate or to the seminal vesicles. Stage T4 tumors have spread to organs near the prostate, such as the bladder.

Stage N+ or M+

Cancer has spread to pelvic lymph nodes (N+) or to lymph nodes, organs, or bones distant from the prostate (M+).

From FDA *Consumer Magazine* (September-October1998).

Expanded Summary of Staging Systems	Whitmore-Jewett System	TNN System
In the earliest stage, prostate cancer can't be felt during a DRE. It is said to be found "incidentally"— during BPH surgery. Biopsied tissue at this stage is less than 5 percent cancerous. Because it is confined to the prostate, small, and low-grade, some doctors recommend "watchful waiting" rather than curative treatment.	A1	T1a
The cancer is not *palpable* (it can't be felt during a DRE) and is found incidentally, during BPH surgery. More than 5 percent of the biopsied tissue is cancerous.	A2	T1b
The cancer is not palpable, but the PSA is elevated and cancer may be found in samples from a needle biopsy.	A3	T1c
Cancer is felt during DRE but is a small nodule confined to less than half of one side of the prostate.	B1N	T2a
Cancer is palpable during DRE and is found in more than half of one side.	B1	T2b
Cancer is palpable during DRE and is found in both lobes, but there's no evidence that it has spread beyond the prostate.	B2	T2c
Cancer occupies one side and is growing outside the capsule.	C1	T3a
Cancer is in both sides and is growing outside the prostate.	C1	T3b
Cancer has spread to the seminal vesicles.	C2	T3c
Cancer has spread to the bladder neck, rectum, or external sphincter, or all three.	C2	T4a
Cancer has spread to other areas in the pelvis.	C2	T4b
There is no cancer found in the lymph nodes.	---	N0
2 cm or a smaller amount of cancer has spread to lymph nodes.	D1	N1 (N+)
2 to 5 cm of cancer has spread to lymph nodes.	D1	N2 (N+)
5 cm or a greater amount of cancer has spread to lymph nodes.	D1	N3 (N+)
Cancer has not spread beyond pelvic tissues and lymph nodes.	---	M0
Cancer has metastasized beyond the pelvis to bones and perhaps other areas.	D2	M1 (M+)

Summary of Treatments
for Prostate Cancer

Prostatectomy

A prostatectomy involves surgically removing the prostate gland and cancer from nearby areas to which the cancer has spread. It is most often used during the cancer's early stages (Stages Tl and T2), when prostate cancer is located only within the prostate. Surgery may help prevent further spread of the cancer. If the cancer is small and located exclusively within the prostate, the surgery may cure the disease.

Advantages: Prostatectomy is a one-time procedure that may cure prostate cancer in its early stages and may help extend life in the later stages.

Disadvantages: Prostatectomy is a major operation that requires hospitalization and can produce side effects, including impotence, incontinence, and narrowing of the urethra, which can make urination difficult. Impotence occurs in a high percentage of patients. In recent years, however, the percentage of men with impotence following surgery has decreased because of a new nerve sparing surgical technique. Permanent incontinence occurs in only a small percentage of patients but it may take some time after the surgery for a patient to regain urinary control

Radiation Therapy

Radiation therapy uses high-energy rays to kill prostate cancer cells, shrink tumors, or prevent cancer cells from dividing and spreading. Because the rays cannot be directed perfectly, they may damage both cancer cells and healthy cells nearby. If the dose of radiation is small and spread out over time, however, the healthy cells are able to recover and survive, and the cancer cells eventually die.

Radiation therapy is usually used when prostate cancer has not spread beyond the prostate (Stages TI-T2). It can help prevent the cancer from spreading further. Like surgery, radiation therapy works best when the cancer is located in a small area. In early stages of prostate cancer, radiation therapy may cure the disease. Radiation therapy may also be used alone or in combination with hormone therapy when cancer cells have spread beyond the prostate to the pelvic area (Stages T3-T4) and for pain relief in prostate cancer that is no longer responding to hormone therapy and has spread to the bones (Stage M+).

There are several ways in which the high-energy rays can be delivered.

External Beam Radiation Therapy

External beam refers to the fact that the radiation therapy is generated and administered by a machine outside of the patients body, as opposed to implants which either temporarily or permanently place radioactive sources within the body. The radiation is typically given in brief sessions, usually one session each weekday for several weeks. External beam therapy include x-ray therapy and Cobalt 60 gamma ray therapy.

CT Conformal Beam Radiation Therapy and Intensity Modulated RadiationTherapy

Both of these are a form of external beam radiation treatment. the goal of which is to shape the beam in three dimensions to the shape of the prostate so that the majority of radiation is given to the tumor and not to the surrounding normal tissue. It is this unique ability to conform a beam to a specific tumor or target which sets it apart from traditional forms of external beam radiotherapy.

Brachytherapy (Seed Implants)

In internal radiation therapy (brachytherapy), the rays come from tiny radioactive seeds inserted directly into the prostate. The seeds are inserted while the patient is under anesthesia; they are too small to cause discomfort. They give off rays continually for about a year and remain safely in place for the rest of a person's life. Internal radiation therapy does not make the patient radioactive.

Another form of internal radiation is delivered by injection and is used to control bone pain in patients with metastasized (Stage M+) prostate cancer that no longer responds to hormone therapy. Radioactive compounds have been found that go directly to the bone and may give dramatic pain relief to many patients with discomfort.

Advantages: With radiation therapy, the patient avoids major surgery. Radiation therapy may cure prostate cancer in its early stages and may help extend life in later stages. It rarely causes loss of urinary control, and it leads to impotence less frequently than does surgery. New injectable radioactive compounds, such as those containing radioactive strontium, can provide pain relief from cancer that has spread to the bone. These new compounds have fewer side effects than do the radioactive phosphorous compounds that have been available for many years.

Disadvantages: Radiation therapy can cause a variety of side effects. Most of these are minor and disappear after therapy stops. These side effects include tiredness, skin reactions in the treated areas, frequent and painful urination, upset stomach, diarrhea, and rectal irritation or bleeding. When radiation therapy is provided by an external machine, it can cause later development of impotence in some patients. Internal radiation therapy causes impotence less often, but may be associated with decreased white blood cell and platelet counts. Radiation therapy is usually a one time only treatment since there is a limit to how much total radiation can be given. Cancer recurrences after radiation therapy may be difficult to treat since both surgery and cryosurgery have much higher complication rates when following radiation.

Cryotherapy / Cryoablation

Targeted cryoablation of the prostate, freezing of prostate cancer tissue, is a minimally invasive therapy involving ultrasound-guided placement of several probes into the prostate. Rapid cooling at the probe tips (using Argon gas) results in immediate cancer cell death with pinpoint accuracy. Recent advances make it safe and effective, especially for men who don't want or can't have surgery or radiation. It may also be very effective for men who are at high risk of having small amounts of cancer just outside the prostate or who have an aggressive tumor (Gleason grade 7or greater). It is FDA-cleared and fully Medicare-approved for primary and salvage treatment of localized prostate cancer with a 89-92 percent success rate in 7-8 year studies.

The procedure is performed under either a spinal (epidural) or general anesthesia. Under ultrasound guidance, slender probes about the size of small knitting needles enter the prostate through tiny holes in the perineum (the skin between the scrotum and the rectum). The probes deliver lethally cold temperatures to cancer cells in two or more freeze-thaw cycles. Thermocouples and a urethral warming device protect healthy tissue from damage. The procedure usually takes an hour and a half or less. Patients go home the day of or morning after.

Cryosurgery is most often suggested for localized or locally advanced disease (T1-T3) or as salvage therapy after any type of failed radiation treatment (recurrence.) It can be combined with hormonal therapy to downsize the gland prior to freezing. When cancer is confined to the prostate or just outside of it, cryo has the potential to cure the disease. With promising improvements in potency rates, cryoablation may be a desirable alternative to major surgery, or to radiation treatments that may diminish potency over time.

Advantages: Avoids major surgery. Less likely to cause urinary tract damage, obstructions, or bowel difficulties than radiation. Patients often fully recover within days. Highest negative biopsy rate at 1, 5 and 7 years of all prostate cancer treatments. Repeatable if necessary.

Disadvantages: Side effects similar to surgery and radiation historically include impotence (22-95 percent), incontinence (1-5 percent), and fistula (less than 1 percent). Recent technology advances and the development of nerve sparing cryo promise significant improvements in potency results.

Hormone Therapy

Hormone therapy is most commonly used to treat cancer that has spread (metastasized) outside the pelvic area (Stages N+ and M+). Two types of hormone therapy can be used: surgical removal of the testicles, which produce male hormones, or drugs that prevent the production or block the action of testosterone and other male hormones. Hormone therapy cannot cure prostate cancer. Instead, it slows the cancer's growth and reduces the size of the tumor or tumors.

Hormone therapy in combination with radiation therapy or surgery is also used in advanced stages of cancer when the disease has spread locally beyond the prostate (Stages T3-T4). This therapy helps extend life and relieve symptoms. When the cancer has spread beyond the prostate, complete surgical removal of the prostate is not common. In patients with early-stage cancer (Stage T2), hormone therapy may be used in combination with radiation therapy. A short course of hormone therapy can also be used prior to surgery to reduce the size of the prostate and make it easier to remove.

The primary strategy of hormone therapy is to decrease the production of testosterone by the testicles. Regardless of the method of hormone therapy, however, the decrease in testosterone can result in certain side effects. These commonly include hot flashes, a loss of sexual desire, and impotence. Osteoporosis may be seen in men on long-term hormone manipulation.

Orchiectomy

An operation called orchiectomy removes the testicles, which produce 95 percent of the body's testosterone.

Advantages: Orchiectomy is an effective procedure that is relatively simple and performed only once. Often, the patient is given a local anesthetic and is allowed to go home the same day as surgery.

Disadvantages: Orchiectomy is a surgical procedure, and many patients prefer a nonsurgical option if it will work as well. Many men also find it difficult to accept this type of surgery. Depending on the kind of anesthesia used, there may be special risks in certain types of patients. Orciectomy may in some cases require hospitalization, and it is not reversible.

Estrogen Therapy

Although not used much anymore, the female hormone estrogen reduces the production of testosterone by the testicles. The most commonly used estrogen in prostate cancer is diethylstilbestrol, or DES. This may be used as a second line therapy after other testosterone limiting therapies have failed.

Advantages: Estrogen therapy is simple and involves taking a pill. Unlike orchiectomy, estrogen therapy does not involve removal of the testicles, and its effects can be reversed.

Disadvantages: Estrogen therapy produces various side effects of its own. Estrogens can cause water retention, embarrassing breast growth and tenderness, and symptoms such as stomach upset, nausea, and vomiting. In addition, even low doses of estrogen may significantly increase the risk of heart and blood vessel problems.

LHRH Therapy

A drug called a luteinizing hormone-releasing hormone analogue (or an LHRH analogue) leads to a drop in testosterone. Taking an LHRH analogue works just as well as removal of the testicles but does not involve surgery. Currently available LHRH analogues are Zoladex and and Lupron.

Advantages: Administering LHRH analogue therapy is simple; it involves an injection every 28 days or every 12 weeks. Treatment with LHRH analogues is as effective as orciectomy, but it does not require surgical removal of the testicles. It also avoids the side effects of estrogen therapy.

Disadvantages: In a small percentage of patients, LHRH analogue therapy may cause a brief rise in cancer symptoms, such as bone pain, before the testosterone level begins to fall. This pain may be eased by the use of a pain reliever (such as aspirin or acetaminophen) or an antiandrogen drug, which is discussed next.

Antiandrogen Therapy

This therapy involves the use of a drug that blocks the action of male hormones. Such a drug is called an antiandrogen. Antiandrogen drugs are used in combination with LHRH analogue therapy. This combination therapy is commonly known as maximal androgen blockade (MAB) or combined hormonal therapy (CHT). The currently available antiandrogens include Casodex, Eulexin, and Viadur, a unique once-yearly implant.

Advantages: Ongoing clinical trials suggest that men treated with MAB therapy live longer than men treated with LHRH analogue therapy alone. The combined use of an LHRH analogue and an antiandrogen can also be of benefit before or after prostate surgery or radiation therapy.

Disadvantages: Antiandrogens may cause gynecomastia (breast enlargement), breast tenderness, hot flushes/hot flashes and loss of libido. Other possible side effects may also include diarrhea, nausea, vomiting, and liver injury.

Chemotherapy

Chemotherapy is the use of powerful toxic drugs to attack cancer cells. The drugs circulate throughout the body in the bloodstream and kill any rapidly growing cells, including healthy ones. To destroy cancer cells while minimizing the harm to healthy ones, the drugs are carefully controlled in dosage and frequency.

Chemotherapy is generally reserved for patients with advanced stage cancer (Stage M+) that no longer responds to hormonal therapy. Chemotherapy drugs do not work well in many men with prostate cancer.

There are many different chemotherapy drugs, each with its own strengths and weaknesses. Often the drugs are used in combination with one another. EmCyt (estramustine phosphate) is a frequently used chemotherapy drug in prostate cancer. Any patient who has evidence of failing hormonal therapy should see a medical oncologist to find out about the latest chemotherapy approaches.

Advantages: Chemotherapy drugs provide an additional means of relieving the symptoms of advanced prostate cancer.

Disadvantages: Because the drugs circulate widely throughout the body and affect healthy as well as cancerous cells, they produce many side effects. These include hair loss, nausea, vomiting, diarrhea, lowered blood counts, reduced ability of the blood to clot, and an increased risk of infection. Most of the side effects disappear when the drugs are stopped. (Hair grows back when chemotherapy is stopped.)

Watchful Waiting

For some patients and certain stages of prostate cancer, the recommended treatment may simply be to "watch and wait," at least in the short term. This means that you won't receive any immediate therapy. Instead, your doctor will monitor the cancer by performing routine DRE and PSA tests. Watchful waiting may be used when prostate cancer is diagnosed at a very early stage or is not expected to progress quickly enough to begin using therapy. Watchful waiting may also be used if a patient is not expected to tolerate other therapy due to other adverse health conditions.

Treatment Summary Courtesy of US TOO International, Inc.

Resources

Prostate Cancer Foundation

1250 Fourth St.
Santa Monica, CA 90401
1-800-757-CURE
(310) 570-4700
www.prostatecancerfoundation.org

The Prostate Cancer Foundation is the world's largest philanthropy supporting prostate cancer research. PCF was founded in 1993 to find better treatments and a cure for advanced prostate cancer. PCF reaches out to private industry, the patient advocacy community, and government research institutions, and has established a system that encourages collaboration, reduces bureaucracy, and speeds the process of discovery. Web site topics include prostate cancer screening, treatment options, risk factors, exercises, personal stories, support groups, financial resources, publications, suggested reading, and news.

American Urological Association

1000 Corporate Blvd.
Linthicum, MD 21090
1-866-746-4282
www.urologyhealth.org

Made up of 13,000 members, this organization strives to keep urologists current on the latest research and best practices in the field of urology. The site also offers patient information, including how prostate cancer is diagnosed and treatment options—surgery, radiation, cryosurgery, chemotherapy, and hormonal therapy. The site also has a "Find a Urologist" feature.

American Foundation for Urologic Disease

1000 Corporate Boulevard
Suite 410
Linthicum, MD 21090
(410) 689-3990
1-800-828-7866
www.afud.org

The foundation is a charitable organization that raises funds for research, lay education, and patient advocacy for the prevention, detection, management, and cure of urologic disease. The foundation's six health councils provide educational materials and international awareness programs about urologic diseases and conditions for the general public and health care providers. The foundation operates the Web site www.prostatehealth.com, with information about prostate conditions, symptoms, diagnosis, and treatment.

National Prostate Cancer Coalition

1154 15˘ Street NW
Washington, D.C. 20005
(202) 463-9455
www.pcacoalition.org

Founded in 1996, the NPCC is an advocacy organization comprised of cancer survivors, doctors, researchers, activists, and other advocate organizations. It strives to create greater public education about prostate cancer in order to detect it early. The organization also reaches out to at-risk and underserved communities by offering free prostate cancer screenings in its mobile clinics.

American Prostate Society

188 Ridge Road
Hanover, MD 21076
(410) 859-3735
www.ameripros.org

This support organization offers online information, including that on the basics of prostate cancer, treatment, and impotence. The organization publishes a quarterly newsletter, which carries updates on the latest treatments available for prostate cancer.

National Kidney and Urologic Diseases Clearinghouse

3 Information Way
Bethesda, MD 20892-3580
(800) 891-5390 or (301) 654-4415
www.kidney.niddk.nih.gov

A service of the National Institutes of Health, this organization provides information about diseases of the kidneys and urological system to patients, their families, health care professionals, and the public. The organization estimates that between 15 and 30 million men experience some form of erectile dysfunction (ED), and offers educational information about ED, how it is diagnosed, and treatment options.

National Association for Continence

P.O. Box 1019
Charleston, SC 29402
(800) BLADDER or (843) 377-0900
www.nafc.org

The goal of this organization is to be a source of information for the 25 million Americans who are affected by incontinence. The Web site offers facts on causes of incontinence, types of incontinence, treatment options, and answers to frequently asked questions.

American Cancer Society

15999 Clifton Road NE
Atlanta, GA 30329-4251
1-800-ACS-2345 (1-800-227-2345)
www.cancer.org

The nation's largest private, not-for-profit source of funds for scientists studying cancer has more than two million volunteers and 3,400 local units working to eliminate cancer as a major health problem through prevention, research, education, patient services, advocacy, and rehabilitation.

National Cancer Institute

Suite 3036A
6116 Executive Boulevard, MSC8322
1-800-4-CANCER (1-800-422-6237)
Bethesda, MD 20892-8322
www.cancer.gov

Part of the National Institutes of Health, The National Cancer Institute coordinates the National Cancer Program, which conducts and supports research, training, health information dissemination, and other programs regarding the cause, diagnosis, prevention, and treatment of cancer, rehabilitation from cancer, and the continuing care of cancer patients and their families.

Cancer Care, Inc.

275 7ᵗ Ave.
New York, NY 10001
Phone: 212-302-2400 (800-813-HOPE)
www.cancercare.org

A nonprofit organization since 1994, Cancer Care offers emotional support, information, and practical help to people with all types of cancer and their loved ones. All services are free. Oncology social workers are available for phone consultations in which they provide emotional counseling and support. Cancer Care also offers educational seminars, teleconferences, and referrals to other services.

The Cancer Information Service (CIS)

National Institutes of Health
Bethesda, MD 20892-2580
Phone: 301-496-4000
1-800-4-CANCER (800-422-6237)
www.cancernet.nci.nih.gov

The National Cancer Institute is part of the National Institutes of Health and is the federal government's principal agency for cancer research and control. The CIS offers free written material and information about treatment, support services, medical facilities, second opinion centers, and clinical trials. Trained information specialists answer cancer-related questions.

OncoLink

The University of Pennsylvania Medical Center
3400 Spruce Street – 2 Donner
Philadelphia, PA 19104
www.oncolink.upenn.edu

Maintained by the University of Pennsylvania, OncoLink's mission is to help cancer patients, families, health care professionals, and the general public receive accurate cancer-related information at no charge. OncoLink offers comprehensive information about specific types of cancer, updates on cancer treatments, and news about research advances. The information (updated every day) is provided at various levels, from introductory to in-depth.

National Coalition for Cancer Survivorship

1010 Wayne Avenue
Suite 770
Silver Spring, MD 20910
(301) 650-9127
www.canceradvocacy.org

The only survivor-led advocacy organization working exclusively on behalf of people with all types of cancer and their families, the NCCS is dedicated to ensuring high-quality cancer care for all Americans.

MEDLINEplus

The U.S. National Library of Medicine
8600 Rockville Pike
Bethesda, MD 20894
www.nlm.nih.gov/medlineplus

Produced by the U.S. National Library of Medicine, MEDLINEplus indexes articles from more than 3,500 medical journals. The service is aimed primarily at scientists and health professionals, but MEDLINEplus is written for consumers.

Radiologyinfo.org

www.radiologyinfo.org

This public information Web site was developed and funded by the American College of Radiology (ACR) and the Radiological Society of North America

(RSNA). It describes dozens of diagnostic and interventional uses of radiation, as well as radiation therapy. The site also includes a thorough description of cryotherapy.

Man to Man

American Cancer Society
15999 Clifton Road NE

Atlanta, GA 30329-4251
1-800-ACS-2345
www.cancer.org

A program of the American Cancer Society, Man to Man offers education, information, sharing and emotional support to meet the challenge of living with prostate cancer. The program helps men cope with prostate cancer by providing community-based education and support to patients and their family members. Activities include community education, a newsletter, outreach to high-risk groups such as African American men, collaboration with health care providers, and free monthly meetings. Local programs may also include one-to-one visitation with a prostate cancer survivor. Meetings are open to spouses and caregivers.

Us Too!

5003 Fairview Avenue
Downers Grove, IL 60515
(630) 795-1002
Support Hotline: 1-800-80-US TOO! (1-800-808-7866)
www.ustoo.org

This not-for-profit organization provides information, counseling, and educational meetings to help men with prostate disease (and their spouses or partners) make decisions about their treatment with confidence and support.

Prostate Pointers

NexCura, Inc.
1725 Westlake Avenue North
Suite 300
Seattle, WA 98109
206-270-0225
www.prostatepointers.org

This inclusive site offers a full spectrum of information about prostate cancer and general problems of the prostate. Topics include libraries, journals, newsletters, and tapes; clinical trials; financial assistance; hospitals, labs, and doctors; impotence and incontinence; news; patient advocacy; recipes; humor; and much more.

Cryocare Prostate Cancer Advocates

www.cryocarepca.org

877-PCA-CRYO (722-2796)

Email: info@cryocarepca.org

This site is dedicated to providing information about cyrosurgery for prostate cancer. The site offers information about how cyrosurgery works, patient stories, a physician locator, recent news about prostate cancer treatment, and a discussion forum.

Phoenix5.org

This web site was developed by prostate cancer survivor Robert Vaughn Young, who was diagnosed in 1999 at age 61. He designed the site to help educate and support men with prostate cancer and their companions. The web site contains information and illustrations about prostate cancer, treatment options, and side effects, along with links to other resources, including state-by-state contacts for support groups and phone list.

Yoursurgery.com

www.yoursurgery.com

This web site seeks to empower and educate patients by providing a comprehensive library of surgical procedures presented in an easy-to-understand format. Designed to be an additional and complementary source of information to a doctor's care, the site offers a basis for patients' questions to their physicians. Each surgery topic has an overview. There's a small cost to view details on anatomy, pathology, examination, testing, indications for surgery, description of the surgical procedure, complications, and after care.

Glossary

A

acute bacterial prostatitis: a sudden severe prostate infection caused by bacteria.

adjuvant therapy: a treatment added to the primary treatment.

adrenal glands: a pair of small glands, one on top of each kidney, that produce small amounts of the male hormone testosterone.

agonist: a drug that simulates physiologic activity at cell receptors stimulated by naturally occurring substances.

alpha-adrenergic agonists: vasoconstrictors (substances that constrict the blood vessels); decongestants.

anastomosis: surgical reattachment of the urethra to the bladder neck after prostatectomy.

androgen blockade: therapy used to eliminate male sex hormones in the body.

androgen deprivation: a treatment that prevents male hormones, principally testosterone, from feeding prostate cancer cells.

androgen-independent cancer: a prostate malignancy that does not depend on male hormones to grow and divide.

androgens: male hormones, including testosterone.

anemia: low red blood cell count.

angiogenesis: the growth of blood vessels.

antagonist: in medicine, a substance that blocks the action of a drug, hormone, or cell.

antiandrogen: a substance that saturates androgen receptors in the prostate and blocks access of testosterone and DHT to those receptors.

anticholinergic agents: drugs that block the neurotransmitter acetylcholine. May be used for urinary urgency.

antibody: substances the body produces to defend against disease.

antioxidants: chemicals (including nutrients such as vitamins A, C, and E) that reduce or prevent oxidation, especially within tissues.

apoptosis: the normal cell death and replacement process.

atypia: variation (indicating disease) in the appearance of the centers of body cells as viewed under a microscope. See also *prostatic intraepithelial neuroplasia (PIN)*.

autologous donation: giving your own blood to be used if you need a transfusion during or after surgery.

B

B-mode acquisition and targeting (BAT): an ultrasound positioning system used in the radiation treatment of prostate cancer to localize targets that may move from one treatment day to the next.

benign: in medicine, noncancerous.

benign prostatic hyperplasia (BPH): prostate enlargement caused by growth of tissue surrounding the urethra.

beta carotene: a nutrient related to vitamin A that is found in dark green and dark yellow fruits and vegetables.

biomarkers: naturally occurring body substances whose fluctuations sometimes indicate cancer.

biopsy: removal of a sample of body tissue for pathological examination.

bisphosphonates: a class of drugs used to prevent or treat osteoporosis.

bone marrow: the soft, spongy centers of large bones where blood cells are made.

bone scan: an imaging study that creates images of bones on a computer screen for diagnosis.

brachytherapy: a procedure in which radioactive seeds are implanted in the body to kill cancer cells.

C

cancer: disease characterized by uncontrolled growth and spread of abnormal cells.

castration level: little or no measurable PSA, as would be achieved by surgical castration.

CAT scan: computerized axial tomography. See *computerized tomography scan*.

central zone: refers to the prostate gland's muscular central zone, which prevents semen from backing up into the bladder during ejaculation.

chemical castration: the use of drugs to reduce testosterone to the level that would be achieved with orchiectomy.

chemotherapy: treatment with anticancer drugs.

chronic bacterial prostatitis: persistent and recurrent inflammation of the prostate caused by bacteria.

Cialis: a PDE-5 inhibitor used to treat impotence and erectile dysfunction; generic, tadalafil.

clinical stage: the suspected extent of cancer's spread using evidence gathered from pretreatment testing. See *pathologic stage; stage*.

colony stimulating factors: drugs that promote white blood cell production.

colostomy: a surgical procedure in which the large intestine is routed to an opening in the body through which fecal waste passes to an external bag.

computerized tomography scan (CT or CAT scan): a diagnostic method that uses computerized X-ray images to create a three-dimensional picture of an internal part of the body.

conformal EBRT: a type of external beam radiation therapy in which the radiation beams are more precisely targeted at a patient's tumor than is the case in conventional EBRT.

continence: in medicine, voluntary control over urination and defecation.

corpora cavernosa: the two parallel chambers of the penis that fill with blood to produce an erection.

corpus spongiosum: a central chamber in the penis through which the urethra passes.

cryoablation: destruction of diseased or damaged tissue by freezing.

cryolumpectomy: a procedure in which supercooled cryoprobes are used to destroy a tumor and a minimal amount of surrounding tissue rather than the entire gland in which the tumor resides.

cryoprobes: supercooled instruments used in cryotherapy.

cryosurgery: see *cryoablation*.

cryotherapy: a medical treatment that destroys abnormal tissues by freezing.

CT scan: see *computerized tomography scan*.

D

debulking: in oncology, reducing the size of a tumor with one treatment, such as hormone therapy or chemotherapy, to facilitate another treatment, such as radiation, cryoablation, or surgery.

deep venous thrombosis: blood clots in the deep veins of the legs.

DEH: see *diethylstilbestrol.*

Denonvillier's fascia: a thin sheet of tissue that separates the prostate and the rectum.

DHT: see *dihydrotestosterone.*

diethylstilbestrol (DES): a form of estrogen.

differentiated: in pathology, a term applied to cells with distinct borders and centers.

diffuse: widespread, scattered, or dispersed.

digital rectal examination (DRE): a diagnostic procedure in which a doctor inserts a gloved, lubricated finger into a man's rectum and feels through the back rectal wall for abnormalities.

dihydrotestosterone (DHT): a potent male hormone to which testosterone is converted in the prostate.

DRE: see *digital rectal examination.*

E

EBRT: see *external beam radiation therapy.*

ejaculatory duct: a channel leading from the seminal vesicle and the vas deferens through the prostate that carries semen out of the body at the time of ejaculation.

endoscope: a long, slender medical instrument equipped with a small camera for examining the interior of an organ or performing surgery.

epididymis: a thin, tightly coiled tube that carries sperm from the testicle to the vas deferens.

epidural: the space between the wall of the spinal canal and the covering of the spinal cord; an anesthetic injection or infusion into this space.

estrogen: a sex hormone that regulates women's reproduction, sometimes used as hormone therapy to treat prostate cancer in men.

external beam radiation therapy (EBRT; XRT): a procedure that uses radiation to destroy cancer from outside the body.

extravasation injury: damage that occurs around the injection site when chemotherapy drugs leak into nearby tissues.

F

Foley catheter: an indwelling catheter—a tube usually inserted for the removal of body waste—the remains in the urethra and bladder until removed.

follicle-stimulating hormone (FSH): a substance that stimulates the testicles to produce testosterone.

free PSA: protein specific antigens that circulate in the blood and are not attached to protein molecules.

free radicals: oxidants; unstable high-energy particles in the body that damage cells.

G

Gleason score: a number between 2 and 10 in a system of grading prostate cancer cells. The lower the number, the closer to normal the cells appear. In general, the higher the number, the more aggressive the tumor.

grade: in oncology, a measure of tumor cells' abnormality and aggressiveness.

granulocytopenia: low white blood cell count.

gynecomastia: breast enlargement and tenderness in men.

H

hematospermia: blood in the semen.

hematuria: blood in the urine.

high-dose-rate implantation (HDR): a brachytherapy procedure in which very high-energy radioactive wires are implanted, left in the body for a short time, then removed.

hormone therapy: in prostate cancer, a treatment whose purpose is to block the body's production, circulation, or absorption of testosterone.

hyperplasia: a benign growth, a thickening or overgrowth of cells.

I

immobilization device: a form-fitting apparatus that helps patients lie perfectly still during external beam radiation therapy.

impotence: the inability to have an erection.

IMRT: see *intensity-modulated radiation therapy.*

incontinence: see *urinary incontinence.*

infusion: in medicine, a method of introducing ("dripping") fluids, including drugs, into the bloodstream.

intensity-modulated radiation therapy (IMRT): in external beam radiation therapy, a technique using multiple small beams that come together to form a single conformal radiation beam.

K

Kegel exercises: a type of muscle training that involves systematically tightening and releasing the urinary sphincter to control the flow of urine.

L

laparoscope: an endoscope (a thin, camera-equipped medical instrument) inserted through a small incision in the abdomen for examination or surgery.

laparoscopic pelvic lymphadenectomy: removal of lymph nodes, using a laparoscope, for pathological examination.

Levitra: a PDE-5 inhibitor used to treat erectile dysfunction or impotence; generic, vardenafil.

LHRH: see *luteinizing hormone releasing hormone.*

LHRH agonist: a substance that tells the pituitary gland to stop producing LHRH.

linear accelerator: a high-energy X-ray treatment machine.

lumpectomy: surgical removal of a tumor and a minimal amount of surrounding tissue rather than the entire gland in which the tumor resides.

luteinizing hormone releasing hormone (LHRH): a substance that stimulates the pituitary gland to release luteinizing hormone.

luteinizing hormone (LH): a substance that stimulates the testicles to produce testosterone.

lycopene: a red pigment (a form of carotenoid) that gives tomatoes their red color and that may help prevent prostate cancer.

lymph: thin clear fluid containing white blood cells that travels through the body's lymphatic system and helps fight infection and disease.

lymphadenectomy: a procedure in which lymph nodes are removed from the body to be examined for cancer.

M

magnetic resonance imaging (MRI): a noninvasive procedure that creates a two-dimensional picture of an internal organ or structure. Magnetic resonance imaging, unlike computerized tomography and X-rays, for example, does not involve radiation.

malignant: in medicine, cancerous.

medical castration: see *chemical castration.*

metastases: cancerous tumors that spread from the original site.

metastasize: spread, as cancer cells.

minilap: see *minilaparotomy staging pelvic lymphadenectomy.*

minilaparotomy staging pelvic lymphadenectomy: a surgical procedure that takes place immediately before retropubic radical prostatectomy. A surgeon removes pelvic lymph nodes through a small incision. If they are found to contain cancer, the prostatectomy is generally canceled.

MRI: see *magnetic resonance imaging.*

multifocal prostate cancer: malignant tumors at several sites within the prostate.

N

nanogram: one billionth of a gram.

needle biopsy: removal of suspected cancer cells through a hollow needle (rather than during a surgical procedure).

neoadjuvant therapy: a treatment given before the primary treatment.

nerve-sparing prostatectomy: surgical removal of the prostate gland that leaves one or both nearby neurovascular bundles intact.

neuropathy: nerve damage expressed as tingling or loss of sensation in the hands or feet.

neurovascular bundles: clusters of nerves near the prostate that enable men to have erections.

neutropenia: low white blood cell count.

nonbacterial prostatitis: inflammation of the prostate from an unknown cause.

O

orchiectomy: surgical castration (removal of the testicles).

organ-confined: of cancer, a tumor or tumors that have not breached the original site.

osteoporosis: a condition of decreased bone mass. This leads to fragile bones which are at an increased risk for fractures.

overflow incontinence: urine leakage that occurs when normal urine flow is blocked and the bladder is always full.

oxidants: see *free radicals.*

P

palliative: used to relieve symptoms rather than cure the underlying illness.

Partin Tables: a tool that uses PSA, clinical stage, and Gleason score to predict how a prostate cancer is likely to behave.

pathologic stage: the actual extent to which a cancer has spread as determined by pathological examination of tissue removed during surgery. See *clinical stage; stage.*

pathologist: a medical doctor who specializes in examinating tissue to make a diagnosis.

patient-controlled analgesia (PCA pump): a pump system for self-administering pain medication. Though patients control their own dosages, the system has safeguards against dosing too much or too often.

PCA pump: see *patient-controlled analgesia.*

PDE-5 inhibitors: drugs used to treat erectile dysfunction and impotence.

pelvic-floor exercises: see *Kegel exercises.*

percutaneous: through unbroken skin.

perineum: the area between the anus and the scrotum.

peripheral zone: the largest part of the prostate, containing about three-fourths of the glands in the prostate.

permanent seed implant (PSI): the permanent implantation of radioactive seeds in the prostate gland.

PET scan: see *positron emission tomography scan.*

phytoestrogens: naturally occurring estrogen-like compounds found in plants.

PIN: see *prostatic intraepithelial neoplasia.*

pituitary gland: located at the base of the brain, the master gland of the endocrine system.

planning study: preparations made for the delivery of radiation therapy.

pneumatic stockings: devices worn on the legs during and after surgery to improve circulation by repeatedly inflating and deflating.

positive margin: cancer identified at the cut surface (insision) of the prostate after surgical removal.

positron emission tomography (PET) scan: a computerized image of body tissues' metabolic activity to determine the presence of disease.

prostate gland: a firm partly muscular chestnut sized gland in males at the base of the bladder; produces a secretion that is the fluid part of semen.

ProstaScint: a staging tool similar to a bone scan except that it finds "hot spots" in soft tissue rather than bones.

prostate capsule: the membrane that encases the numerous small glands of the prostate.

prostate-specific antigen (PSA): a protein manufactured by the prostate to help liquefy semen. Elevated PSA levels can signal prostate disease.

prostatic intraepithelial neoplasia (PIN): cell abnormalities sometimes described as precancerous. See also *atypia.*

prostatitis: inflammation of the prostate.

PSA: see *prostate-specific antigen.*

PSA velocity: the rate at which PSA levels rise.

pubis: one of the pelvic bones.

pulmonary embolism: a blood clot in the lung.

R

radiation oncologist: a medical doctor who specializes in using radiation to treat cancer.

radical laparoscopic prostatectomy: surgical removal of the prostate through a small abdominal incision using an endoscope.

radical perineal prostatectomy: a surgical procedure in which the prostate is removed through an incision in the perineum.

radical prostatectomy: surgical removal of the prostate, seminal vesicles, and pelvic lymph nodes.

radical retropubic prostatectomy: a surgical procedure in which the prostate seminal vesicles, and pelvic lymph nodes are removed through an incision in the lower abdomen.

radioactive seeds: energy-emitting pellets implanted to kill cancer cells.

radioresistant: of tumors, those that are not easily destroyed by radiation therapy.

S

salvage therapy: in prostate cancer, a follow-up treatment used when the primary treatment has failed to eradicate the disease.

saturation biopsy: a biopsy in which specimens are obtained at 5mm intervals throughout the prostate. Carried out through the perineum under ultrasound guidance.

seed implantation: a procedure in which radioactive seeds are placed in the body to kill cancer cells.

semen: a milky liquid produced by the seminal vesicles to carry sperm out of the body.

seminal fluid: Fluid from the prostate and other sex glands that help transport sperm during orgasm.

seminal vesicles: small organs alongside the prostate that manufacture semen.

sepsis: a serious illness caused by severe infection of the bloodstream by a toxin-producing bacteria, virus, or fungus.

stage: of cancer, the extent to which a tumor has spread from its primary site. See *clinical stage; pathologic stage.*

staging pelvic lymphadenectomy: removal of pelvic lymph nodes to determine whether cancer has spread from the prostate.

stress urinary incontinence: involuntary leakage of urine caused by activity or the sudden movement involved in sneezing, coughing, or laughing.

surgical castration: see *orchiectomy.*

T

3D global mapping biopsy: see *saturation biopsy.*

temporary seed implant: see *high-dose-rate implantation (HDR).*

testes: see *testicles.*

testicles: the principal organs where the male hormone testosterone is produced.

testosterone: the predominant male hormone, responsible for most male-related traits.

thrombocytopenia: low blood platelet level.

TNM staging system: method of classifying malignant tumors with respect to primary tumor, involvement of regional lymph nodes, and presence or absence of metastastes.

transrectal ultrasound (TRUS): an imaging technique in which sound waves produce a "picture" of the prostate and abnormalities it might contain.

transurethral resection of the prostate (TURP): surgery to remove prostate tissue through the urethra to treat benign prostatic hyperplasia.

TRUS: see *transrectal ultrasound.*

tumor: a mass of abnormal cells, which may be malignant (cancerous) or benign (noncancerous).

tumor markers: see *biomarkers*.

TURP: see *transurethral resection of the prostate*.

U

unifocal prostate cancer: a single malignant tumor within the prostate.

ureters: tubes that carry urine from the kidneys to the bladder.

urethra: the duct through which urine leaves the body; also, in males, the genital duct.

urethral stricture: narrowing of the urethra caused by scar tissue that forms after surgery.

urethrorectal fistula: a hole between the digestive and urinary tracts.

urge incontinence: the inability to hold urine long enough to reach a restroom.

urinary bladder: the organ in which urine is stored after leaving the kidneys and before leaving the body.

urinary incontinence: inability to control the leaking of urine from the body.

urinary sphincter: the ring of muscle that contracts to prevent urine from leaking.

urologist: a physician who has special knowledge of the male and female urinary tract and the male reproductive organs.

V

vas deferens: singular form of *vasa deferentia*.

vasa deferentia: the tubes that carry sperm out of the testicles.

vasodilator: a drug that widens blood vessels.

venous access device: a port, under the skin, usually in the chest area, for accessing veins to administer medications intravenously.

viagra: a PDE-5 inhibitor used to treat erectile dysfunction or impotence; generic, sildenafil citrate.

W

Whitmore-Jewett staging system: a method of describing prostate cancer's spread, less commonly used than the TNM staging system.

X

XRT: see *external beam radiation therapy*.

Index

About the Authors

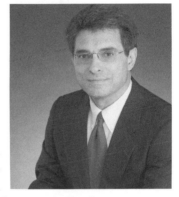

Arthur S. Centeno, M.D.,** is a board-certified urologist in private practice at Urology San Antonio in San Antonio, Texas. He treats prostate cancer patients through surgery, brachytherapy, and cryosurgery.

"I decided I wanted to be a doctor when I was 12 years old and while visiting my grandfather in the hospital. I realized I wanted to help people. My philosophy of medicine has evolved over the years. I have learned it is important that doctors be more than medical technologists—they must also be empathetic to patients and families. This became so clear to me when my wife died of breast cancer three years ago. I teach my medical students that we are dealing with people, not just diseases."

Dr. Centeno is a graduate of the University of Texas Health Science Center in San Antonio, Texas, where he is now a clinical associate professor in the Division of Urology. He completed his surgical internship and residency in urology at the University of Texas Medical Branch in Galveston, Texas, and earned a Master of Medical Sciences degree at that institution's Graduate School of Biomedical Sciences.

Dr. Centeno is a member of the American Urological Association and Sigma Xi Scientific Research Society, and is a Fellow of the American College of Surgeons. He has two children, Rebecca and Everett.

Dr. Centeno may be reached at www.urologysanantonio.com.

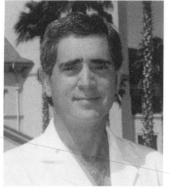

Gary Onik, M.D., is a board-certified radiologist and the director of surgical imaging at Celebration Health Florida Hospital in Orlando, Florida. "I became a radiologist because it was clear to me that the marriage of surgery and imaging was going to open new vistas in the treatment of cancer patients. Our dedication to this concept and our lack of satisfaction with the status quo has definitely resulted in prolonged survival with fewer complications for our patients."

Dr. Onik is widely credited as being the father of ultrasound-guided tumor ablation. He carried out the first ultrasound-guided prostate cancer cryosurgical ablation in the early 1990s.

Dr. Onik received his undergraduate degree from Harvard University and graduated from New York Medical College. He completed his residency in radiology at the University of California–San Francisco. He has also completed fellowships in computeried tomography, ultrasound, and interventional radiology at New England Deaconess Hospital, Harvard Medical School.

The author of four academic medical textbooks, Dr. Onik has also published more than seventy articles in peer-reviewed medical journals. He has won numerous awards for his pioneering work in minimally invasive surgery, including being nominated for the Russ Prize, the highest honor of the National Academy of Engineering in bioengineering. Dr. Onik continues to collaborate in ongoing research with many of the world's experts in prostate cancer.

Dr. Onik may be reached at www.hopeforprostatecancer.com.

Other Consumer Health Titles from Addicus Books
Visit our online catalog at www.AddicusBooks.com

After Mastectomy—Healing Physically and Emotionally *$14.95*

Cancers of the Mouth and Throat—A Patient's Guide to Treatment *$14.95*

Cataracts: A Patient's Guide to Treatment *$14.95*

Colon & Rectal Cancer—A Patient's Guide to Treatment *$14.95*

Coping with Psoriasis—A Patient's Guide to Treatment *$14.95*

Coronary Heart Disease—A Guide to Diagnosis and Treatment *$15.95*

Exercising Through Your Pregnancy *$17.95*

The Fertility Handbook—A Guide to Getting Pregnant *$14.95*

*The Healing Touch—Keeping the Doctor/Patient
   Relationship Alive Under Managed Care* *$9.95*

The Macular Degeneration Source Book *$14.95*

LASIK—A Guide to Laser Vision Correction *$14.95*

Living with P.C.O.S.—Polycystic Ovarian Syndrome *$14.95*

Lung Cancer—A Guide to Treatment & Diagnosis *$14.95*

The Macular Degeneration Source Book *$14.95*

The Non-Surgical Facelift Book—A Guide to Facial Rejuvenation Procedures . *$19.95*

Overcoming Postpartum Depression and Anxiety *$14.95*

A Patient's Guide to Dental Implants *$14.95*

Prescription Drug Addiction—The Hidden Epidemic *$15.95*

Prostate Cancer—A Patient's Guide to Treatment *$14.95*

Simple Changes: The Boomer's Guide to a Healthier, Happier Life *$9.95*

A Simple Guide to Thyroid Disorders *$14.95*

Straight Talk About Breast Cancer—From Diagnosis to Recovery *$14.95*

The Stroke Recovery Book—A Guide for Patients and Families *$14.95*

The Surgery Handbook—A Guide to Understanding Your Operation *$14.95*

Understanding Lumpectomy—A Treatment Guide for Breast Cancer *$14.95*

Understanding Parkinson's Disease—A Self-Help Guide *$14.95*

Organizations, associations, corporations, hospitals, and other groups may qualify for special discounts when ordering more than 24 copies. For more information, please contact the Special Sales Department at Addicus Books. Phone (402) 330-7493. Email: Addicusbks@aol.com

Please send:

_____copies of_____
(Title of book)

at $_____each   TOTAL: _____

Nebraska residents add 5% sales tax   _____

Shipping/Handling
   $4.00 postage for first book.
   $1.10 postage for each additional book   _____

   TOTAL ENCLOSED: _____

Name _____

Address _____

City_____State_____Zip _____

☐ **Visa**   ☐ **MasterCard**   ☐ **American Express**

Credit card number _____Expiration date _____

Order by credit card, personal check or money order. Send to:

Addicus Books
Mail Order Dept.
P.O. Box 45327
Omaha, NE 68145
Or, order **TOLL FREE: 800-352-2873**
or online at
www.AddicusBooks.com